CW00518482

THE HISTORY
OF
DONNINGTON HOSPITAL
A Family Charity

CECILIA MILLSON

Countryside Books
Newbury

Designed by Publicity Plus Partnership, Newbury.
Typeset in Great Britain by
Acorn Bookwork, Salisbury, Wiltshire.
Printed and bound through
MRM (Print Consultants) Ltd., Reading.

CONTENTS

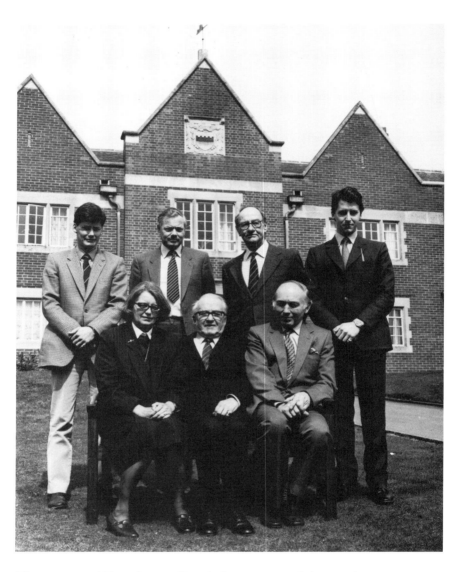

The trustees of Donnington Hospital 1985. From left to right:
BACK ROW: Rupert Hartley Russell, Derek Parkes (Clerk to the Trustees),
Philip Dalton, Robin Hartley Russell.
FRONT ROW: Pam Hartley Russell (Chairman), Derek Hartley Russell
(Patron), Keith Hall (Vice-Chairman).
The other trustees not in the picture are Rev. Richard Capstick, Rev. John
Blick and Dr Gordon Hunter.

The Dawn of the Hospital

For six hundred years the proud gatehouse of Donnington Castle has dominated the surrounding countryside from the top of a windswept hill. Far below, on the banks of the river Lambourn, the twelve almshouses of Donnington Hospital have enjoyed a far more sheltered position, but both gatehouse and hospital owe their existence to the same man – Sir Richard de Abberbury.

The de Abberburys were lords of the manor of Donnington at the end of the thirteenth century and Sir Richard inherited the manor and castle in 1353 from John de Abberbury who was probably his cousin. A man of property in Berkshire, Oxfordshire and Wiltshire, Sir Richard served as a knight in the campaigns of the Black Prince and later became one of the three guardians of his son, Prince Richard. With the death of the Black Prince in 1376 his son became heir to the throne and succeeded his grandfather, Edward III, who died in 1377. The former guardian became the young king's friend and adviser and, in due course, was appointed chamberlain to King Richard's consort, Anne of Bohemia.

In 1386, when Sir Richard wished to extend and crenellate his castle at Donnington, the king was pleased to grant the necessary licence, a privilege only awarded to such nobles deemed worthy of the king's trust in an age of rebellion and unrest. As a result of Richard II's favour the imposing gatehouse was added to the original building and time proved it to be the most formidable part of the castle.

Sir Richard Abberbury suffered for his loyalty to the king when he was expelled from the court in 1388 by the king's opponents, known as the Lords Appellant. By then he was an old man and, sad though he may have been for his royal master's plight, it was probably with relief that he retired to his country estates away from the intrigue of the court. The ageing knight was not recalled when the king reasserted his authority the following year.

Released at last from duties of State the lord of the manor was free to ride out from his castle to enjoy the tranquillity of his riverside meadows and to meditate upon his spiritual well being. Not that he had neglected his religious observances in the past. In 1365 he had obtained a licence to build and endow a chapel in Donnington and had granted lands to the friars of the Holy Cross (or Crutched Friars) in London in 1376 so that two of their order might be sent to officiate in the chapel. But now, as his advancing years weighed heavily upon him, Sir Richard's thoughts turned to most serious matters – the provision for the aged poor of his manor, and the salvation of the king's, his own, and his family's souls.

It was a custom of the period for the wealthy landowners and successful citizens to provide for the sick and aged who, in return, prayed for the well being of their benefactors in this life and for their souls in the life to come. This type of charity fulfilled Sir Richard's needs and he formulated plans for the erection of a hospital to provide homes for twelve poor men and their minister whose daily prayers in the existing chapel would include supplications on behalf of the king, himself and his family. What Sir Richard could never have foreseen was the success of his benefaction six hundred years after his foundation. How proud he would have been to know that to this day his castle gatehouse still stands like a sentinel over the almshouses of Donnington Hospital.

The Foundation of the Hospital

Richard de Abberbury gave two acres of land in Donnington for the erection of his new foundation and made a further gift of the manor of Iffley in Oxfordshire for the maintenance of the alms-houses and their inmates. This manor had been granted to him by Queen Anne in 1383, the grant being for her lifetime. Two years later the king confirmed and extended the grant, giving the manor in fee to Sir Richard who had sold land of his own in earlier years in order to finance the king.

In 1393 the king granted a licence for the foundation of the hospital and his consent to the endowment of the foundation with the manor of Iffley. The following extract from Richard II's grant was quoted by Mr Walter Money in the *Transactions of the Newbury Field Club*, Vol. III, p. 56 (1875–86).
'Know ye that whereas our beloved and faithful Richard Abberbury, Knight, remembering the end of his days, and looking forward to things above, hath proposed newly to found make and establish a certain Hospital or House of certain poor men at his Manor of Donnington, which is held of us as of the honour of Wallingford; there perpetually to attend upon God, and specially for the healthful state of us, and of the same Richard, while we shall live, and for our souls when we shall depart out of this life, and for the souls of our progenitors and heirs, and of the predecessors and heirs of the same Richard, for ever to pray, according to the ordinances of the same Richard on this part to be made; and by the intervention of his licence to give, grant and assign to the same poor men and their successors two acres of land which are parcel of the said Manor of Donnington, for their habitation, and the Manor of Yifteley with its appurtenances for their maintenance. We to the pious intent and wholesome purpose of the aforesaid Richard the eye of our consideration earnestly directing, and in order that we may become partakers in the rewards of so great and so perfect a work of piety and merit – of our special favour, and at the prayer of

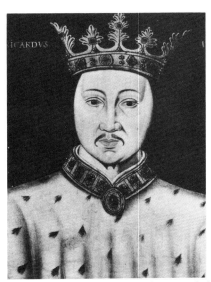

Richard II who granted a licence for the foundation of the Hospital in 1393

the said Richard, have granted and given licence for us and for our heirs aforesaid, so far as in us lies, to the same Richard, to found and establish at his said Manor of Donnington, a certain perpetual house of poor men, of whom one shall be over the others, and be named the Minister of God's Poor House of Donnington, and we grant and assign the Manor of Yifteley with its appurtenances for their maintenance: to hold etc . . .' 'At Westminster, 26th April, 1393' (Translated from Dug. Mon., volvi., p. 715).

With plans for his hospital finally established the founder proceeded to draw up a set of 'Lawes, Statutes and Ordinances' to define the desired administration of the charity and the behaviour and duties required of the almsmen.

> 'Hereafter follow the Lawes Statutes and Ordinances of Sir Richard Abberbury, Kt. founder originall of the Hospitall or Almes House of Donington on the county of Berks by the licence of Richard the Second, King of England, and in the xviith yeare of his reigne.
>
> 1.   Ffirst to the worship of Almighty God and our lady St. Mary and all the holy company of Heaven, Sr. Richard Aberbury, Knight hath here founded an Almeshouse by leave of the King for to last without end for thirteen poor men to keepe under ordinances and statutes (of his own making) whilst that he here lived and for to pray for the

state of Sr. Richard Aberbury his sonne and Alice his Wife, and all his heyres that live and for the soules of Sr. Richard Aberbury Knight, our founder and Anne his wife and all his children that be dead and for the soules that he is due and in debt to pray for and for all Christians.

2. Alsoe he hath ordained that as soon as any man is passed out of this house by way of death, either put out by trespasse making, another shall be chosen by his heyres of his poore tenants either of his servants or some poore man to whom he liketh his almes for to give.

3. Allsoe he hath ordained that he that shall be here Governor and Master Dwelling among them shall be clipped (ycleped – called) Minister to whome all his brethren shall be obedient and bound all the ordinances and statutes for too keepe.

4. Allsoe he hath ordained that if the Minister be passed out of this World that another here amongst us be chosen by our common assent if that there be any person able in manner and in cunning provided and examined before his heyres or else that it be lawfull that his heyres choose one without for the Governall of the house to have, and to rule.

5. Allsoe he hath ordained that every poore man be honest of manners (that is to say) That there be no comon chider, nor fighter, nor Jangler, nor ale-house goer, neither of none yther wise by the which I may be disslandered and the house greatly hindered.

6. Allsoe he hath ordained that none of us shall goe by streets, neither by dores, neither sit by wayes, men's almes for to ask.

7. Allsoe he hath ordained that the Minister and all his brethren that be at home and now goe shall every day heare Masse among his ffreers and every day say fifty paternosters and fifty aves and three Creeds for the lives and soules that be spoken of before.

8. Allsoe he hath ordained that the Minister and all his brethren that shall dwell in his house shall be sworn on the Book anon at their incoming, the statutes to be made and to keepe.

9. Allsoe he hath ordained that none of the brethren from the time of their incoming shall none of their goods or chattels alien nor waste, but spend them in good way at their need, and after their decease and going out turne to the common profit.

10. Allsoe he hath ordained that if there be any of ye brethren that layeth his hands on the Minister violent either els in-obedient and rebell to his lawfull commandments, or else he will not keepe his statutes after the discretion of the Minister, utterly to be put out.

11. Alsoe he hath ordained and given us his manner of Yeftley with all the appurtenances thereto in Oxfordshire, and an annuall rent of twenty six quarters of Wheate a yeare or else therteene marks of Gold for the very value thereof for to depart amongst us in this manner: first to ye Minister three quarters and four bushells of Wheat or else the price assigned; and to every of his brethren a quarter of wheat and seven bushells or the price, delivered at foure termes of the year; and to the Minister and to every one of his brethren each day a peny of the same manner and of profits coming thereof.

12. Allsoe that he hath ordained that the residue which is levyed over be put in a common coffer to treasure for the reparations of this our Almes house and of our manner. The which coffer shall be safe lock'd with three keys, of which keys the minister shall keepe one, they either shall be delivered to two of the brethren which shall be chosen by comon assent and newed every yeare that by virtue of obedience it shall be kept.

13. Allsoe he hath ordained that the Minister every yeare betwixt the feast of St. Michaell and Christmas shall give his full accompts of all things he has received and departed amongst his brethren and also spended in comon profits before one of our Lords' Councell which the lord will assign in presence of all the brethren of the Almes house gathered together; and if it shall be found that the Minister be found in rerage, then he hath ordained that he shall withdraw of half his living unto the time that he hath made amends of all things that he is found guilty in, and if it be found that ye minister be convicted and demed thrice in rerages and within the tenth day after the third warning make none amends he shall be deprived of his office, and another by new election put in his steed and half of the livelide that thus is withdrawn shall be put in the comon treasure in our house needs for to be spended.

14. Allsoe he hath ordained that none of the brethren without license of the minister by the space of a night, neither to noe towne, nor village be so bold, neither so hardy for to goe, and if there be any out of the house three days without leave anone, he shall be put out and an other in his steed sett.

15. Allsoe he hath ordained that if any of us passe hence as by way of Death either for trespasse making, that his portion shall be kept in treasure, of which the minister shall give accompt and of all goods and chattels that liveth after the decease of any of our brethren.

16. Allsoe he hath ordained that if there come any poore man by the way and ask harbour for the love of God that he be received and have a night's lodging and easement of housing and of a bed.

17.   Also he hath ordained for the common profit that there shall be a comon seale to notify covenants that hath bin made or shall be made betwixt us and other men, the which shall be kept in comon Treasure under three keys.

18.   Allsoe he hath ordained that we shall alien no land, neither no part of our Almes house or belonging thereto, neither to our manner of Yeftley in no manner of fee; neither to noe man to let out soe long time by which our place might be alienated away from us. Neither it shall not be lawful to our Lands, nor Tenements for to let to our Tenants and their hyres for terme yf lifes, but be right good sikernes (security), made by good comon counsell. Neither it shall not be lawful to us to bring our Almes house, neither our manner of Yeftley, neither noe part belonging to it in thraldom of percon, neither of charges goeing out of them by which that place might be greatly hindered in paine of perjury and of loosing our places.

19.   Alsoe he hath ordained that every one of us that now in this Almes House be, and that hereafter shall be to come in to live, do know the statutes, and every week (being all gather'd together) shall heare them here read on the fridayes for their colation. And for the Soule that them ordained each man shall say anone after five paternosters and five aves and a Creed. Soe be it.

It seems strange that prayers for the well-being of Richard II were not included in the above statutes, as by the terms of his grant the king obviously assumed that the almsmen would remember him in their daily devotions. Perhaps his erstwhile guardian considered it imprudent to mention Richard by name during these turbulent years of his reign and contented himself that the king's welfare was covered by the phrase 'and for the soules that he is due to pray for and for all Christians'. Richard was deposed in 1399 and a year later died, or was murdered, in Pontefract Castle.

The date of Sir Richard Abberbury's death is not known but it would appear that he was still alive in 1397 as a bequest under the will of John of Gaunt was made to 'Mons. Ric. Abberbury le fils'. This was, no doubt, the son for whom, with Alice his wife, the almsmen were to say daily prayers. Apparently there were no children of this marriage to inherit the manor, and, his father having died sometime during the intervening years, the then Sir Richard Abberbury, together with Alice his wife, sold their estates in Donnington in 1415 to a member of another well known medieval family, Thomas Chaucer, reputedly the son of the poet Geoffrey Chaucer.

The Hospital through Hazardous Years

Thomas Chaucer was a man of considerable standing. By the time he acquired the manor of Donnington he had been Sheriff of Berkshire and Oxfordshire, Constable of the King's Castle of Wallingford and four times Speaker of the House of Commons (1407, 1410, 1411, and 1414). He was Member of Parliament for Oxford and was appointed Chief Butler of England during the reigns of both Henry IV and Henry V. He added to his own considerable estates by marrying Matilda, co-heiress of the Burghersh family, whose Oxfordshire estates included the Manor of Ewelme. Their only child, Alice, was born in 1404 and was betrothed in childhood to Sir John Phelips but he died before she reached the age of twelve years and the young heiress eventually married Thomas Montacute, Earl of Salisbury. This contract was destined to end tragically as the Earl was killed at the siege of Orleans in 1428. Alice then married another powerful nobleman, William de la Pole, Earl of Suffolk, supporter and favourite of Henry VI who rewarded his loyalty by bestowing a dukedom upon him.

The Duke and Duchess of Suffolk visited Donnington and took an interest in the hospital. According to some reports the Duke was responsible for its completion. He was styled as the minister although it seems reasonable to suppose that he left most of the administrative work in the hands of the thirteenth almsman, for his interests were many and his other estates naturally claimed a fair share of the time he could spare from affairs of State.

With the Duchess, Suffolk was particularly interested in her manor of Ewelme which they planned to develop into a model village. The church and manor house were to be rebuilt and, perhaps with the example of Donnington in mind, twelve almshouses were to be erected, but the Duke and Duchess, while providing for the aged, also remembered the young and a school was to be part of their charitable gift to Ewelme. Alas, before their plans came to fruition, Suffolk was murdered on his way to

France. In spite of the beneficent image he presented to Donnington and Ewelme the Duke was extremely unpopular nationally having arranged the marriage between Henry VI and the hated Margaret of Anjou. Furthermore, he was accused of murdering the king's uncle, the Duke of Gloucester, although it was probable that Gloucester's death was from natural causes following the shock of his arrest on a charge of treason. The Duke of Suffolk was arrested by petition of Parliament and sent to the Tower of London. Powerful friends managed to secure his release and the king, in an effort to further his favourite's safety, exiled him to France for five years. The Duke left Ipswich on 3rd May 1450, but his ship was halted on the high seas by his enemies aboard the *Nicholas of the Tower* and he was taken captive and brutally beheaded on the side of the ship.

The Duchess was left to complete the development of Ewelme, a task which occupied the twenty-five years of her widowhood. She is not only remembered for her charitable work but also by the magnificent tomb erected in the church of St Mary at Ewelme. It was probably commissioned by her son, John de la Pole, 2nd Duke of Suffolk. He brought royal connection to his manors by marrying Elizabeth Plantagenet, the sister of Edward IV, but it is not known whether they concerned themselves with the management of Donnington Hospital. Probably they had enough to occupy them with family affairs. Their eldest son, created Earl of Lincoln, was declared the heir to his uncle Richard III, after the death of the Prince of Wales, but with the defeat and death of Richard on Bosworth Field in 1485, Henry VII became king and the Earl of Lincoln was set aside. He supported the imposter Lambert Simnel against Henry and died at the Battle of Stoke in 1487, four years before the death of his father. The second son, Edmund de la Pole, inherited his father's estates but not the Dukedom. Henry VII reduced his status to Earl of Suffolk. Understandably, the Earl was not happy with the new regime and soon showed his dislike of the Tudors with the result that he lost his title by attainder in 1503, together with his estates which passed to the Crown. Donnington Castle and manor, and therefore the hospital, became royal possessions, and the badge of Henry VII (a rose per pale gules and argent crowned or) within the Garter, was seen by Richard Symonds in 1644 in a window of the castle. In 1513, four years after the accession of Henry VIII, the ill-fated

Edmund de la Pole was beheaded in the Tower.

History records the fate of the noble owners of Donnington during the fifteenth century but little is known of the day to day life of the hospital's inhabitants. At the turn of the century Lyson gives us a brief glimpse into the life, or rather the death, of one of the ministers by citing the will of Robert Harre. Bearing the date 1500 it directed that his body should be buried in the new chapel of Jesus on the south side of the church of the Friars of the Holy Cross in Donnington, his two great standards of laten to stand before the altar of Jesus in the said Chapel of Donnington and four candlesticks of laten to stand before the said altar.

On the 20th June 1509, Winstan Brown, squire of the body to Henry VIII, was appointed keeper of the manor and park of Donnington, steward of the lordship, and minister of the king's almshouses at Donnington. But his appointment was but brief for on the 31st July of the same year Sir John Daunce succeeded him at Donnington and remained in office until 1513.

On October 29th of that year Sir William Compton was appointed keeper of the manor and park, bailiff of the lordship, minister of the hospital and steward of the manor of Donnington. However, the following year the king granted the castle, park and manor of Donnington with the hospital and its appurtenances, together with other estates, to his brother-in-law, Charles Brandon, Viscount Lisle, whom he created Duke of Suffolk. During the time the manor belonged to the Duke, Edward Fettiplace of Sandford acted as his keeper and the minister of the hospital, but he was not over zealous in his duties and was blamed for the poor condition of the castle when it was handed back to the Crown in 1535, the Duke having exchanged the manor of Donnington for other properties by arrangement with the king.

Donnington was to see further change in 1538 for the priory did not escape notice during the dissolution of the monastic houses which took place throughout the length and breadth of England during that period. The priory was closed and the remaining friars were given small pensions and turned away to seek some other form of livelihood.

The hospital, not being connected with the priory, was allowed to remain to give shelter to its poor men, although, no doubt, they missed the companionship and counsel which the friars had given them especially as one of the almsmen was to suffer a most cruel punishment for a small offence. Thomas Barrie spread a rumour that the king was dead. Apparently he had reason to believe that he spoke the truth but, unfortunately for him, it was a false rumour. He was taken to Newbury one market day and nailed by his ears to the pillory. At the end of the day he was released by the cutting off of his ears – a dreadful retribution for making a mistake.

The following year (1539) the king gave lie to the rumour in person for he visited Donnington Castle. Perhaps he may even have seen the mutilated old man as he passed by the hospital.

The castle must have pleased the king as he repeated his visit in 1541, no doubt causing much stir in the village and excited, if cautious, chatter among the inhabitants of the hospital.

By an act of 1545 all colleges, free chapels, chantries, hospitals and fraternities with their lands, tenements, and hereditaments were granted to the Crown. Donnington Hospital was described as follows in the Commissioner's Report (*Newbury District Field Club Transactions* Vol. III, p. 60).

'Berks – the Parishe of Donnyngton'
'One hospytall there founded by Walter Abberbury to the intent to have XIII pore men there to continewe for ever, and every one of them to have towards theyr livynge 1d by the daye and one chamber and 12s.6d. in the mone of corne money whych the have accordyngiy. The patron or donor thereof nowe ys in the King's matie. The said hospitall ys nyghe adioyninge to the Castell of Donnynton dystaunte frome the pishe churche of Donnynton half a mile. The value of the lande and posessions apptenynge to the same hospitall £28.16.8d. whereoff ffor the stipent of XIII pore men £19.5s.5d. (*this sum should be £19.15s.5d. as will be found by working out the total*), ffor corne money to the same pore men £8.2s.6d. And so remayneth – 18s.9d. whych ys towarde the repayrynge of the tenemente. Ornaments plate juelles goods and catalle merly appteynynge unto the said hospytall ther ar none for yt ys served wt thornaments of the same church' (Chantry Certificate, Berks, No. 51, P.R.O.)

The Act caused the hospital little, if any disturbance as it was already in royal ownership.

With the death of Henry VIII in 1547 the manor passed to his son, Edward VI. In April 1551 the young king granted it to his half-sister, the Princess Elizabeth, a grant which was to have far-reaching effects on the future of the hospital.

The Re-Foundation
of the Hospital

King Edward VI visited Donnington in September, 1551 and stayed at the Castle for two days during which time he held a Privy Council. The Princess Elizabeth wished to come to her castle during the time of her captivity in the reign of Mary Tudor, but her half sister forbade her that pleasure and it was not until she had succeeded to the throne herself that Elizabeth was able to visit her manor of Donnington.

In 1568 the castle was made ready for a visit by the Sovereign. Repairs were carried out and the old drawbridge was replaced by a new bridge to the gatehouse. New and costly fittings were provided for the interior. The Queen demanded comfortable and splendid lodgings for herself and her courtiers, and judging by the accounts, and orders to the tradespeople of Newbury, it would appear that temporary accommodation was provided for some of her large retinue during the visit.

In 1590 Elizabeth honoured another lady, almost as formidable as the Queen herself, when she appointed Lady Russell as Keeper of Donnington Castle. Perhaps better known as Lady Hoby, the resolute and learned wife of Sir Thomas Hoby of Bisham Abbey, this strong minded lady had married as her second husband, Lord John Russell, son of Frances, fourth Earl of Bedford. Her hopes of becoming a countess were thwarted when her husband predeceased his father, but her pride must have been mollified by the honour of the Donnington appointment. No doubt she was aware of the almshouses lying in the shadow of her castle, even if she had no jurisdiction over their administration.

This was in the hands of various ministers under the patronage of the Queen. In 1559 there was a Thomas Carradine who was followed two years later by Thomas Beke. He, in turn, was succeeded by Thomas Litherland who immediately placed the finances of the hospital in jeopardy by making an improvident lease of Iffley. The next minister, Sir Anthony Ashley, with the

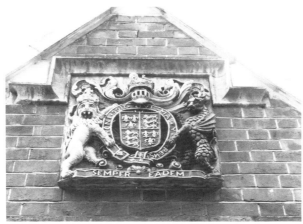

The Stone Arms of Elizabeth I at Donnington

help of the past minister, Thomas Beke, managed to have this unfortunate lease set aside in 1597/8. The court ruled that the hospital was held to be a superstitious hospital, being erected not so much for the relief of the poor as for prayer for souls. As such it was deemed dissolved under the Chantry Act. Therefore, it was decided that there had been no corporation in the eighth year of Elizabeth's reign competent to grant a lease. It was a strange verdict which, although it cancelled the offending lease, it brought into question the very validity of the hospital's existence.

Furthermore the next minister, Thomas Flory, pleaded in 1599 that the rent reserved by the lease made in the eighth year of Elizabeth's reign was £100 too little, that the stipend of the almsmen was only 7d. a week and they were very poor, while the hospital itself was in great decay and ruin.

Dark days indeed for Donnington Hospital. But the following year the tide turned and Queen Elizabeth's interest was aroused, perhaps rather belatedly, so that the future of Sir Richard Abberbury's foundation was ensured for generations to come.

In the year 1600 the Queen wished to express her gratitude to Charles Howard, Earl of Nottingham, for the part he had played in the defeat of the Spanish Armada. She did so by bestowing certain lands upon him which included the lordship and manor of Donnington. The following is an extract from the Grant of the Manor of Donnington dated the fifteenth day of May in the 42nd year of her reign.

'Know ye that we having certain knowledge that our most dear Cousin and Counsellor Charles Earl of Nottingham Baron Howard of Effingham of the most noble order of the Garter Knight hath strenuously and bravely borne himself for some years past as High Admiral of England and more especially hath rendered excellent service to Us and our Kingdom with our Royal ships and Fleet and Army in the Year of our Lord one thousand five hundred and eighty eight under our auspices and by favour of God in Naval battle on the high seas hath overcome the Spanish Fleet prepared to invade our Kingdom although in number the ships of the Spaniards were much more the Duke of Medina Sidonia Supreme Head and Captain General of the Spanish Army being put to flight and the greater part of the Fleet either destroyed or sunk And by gaining that victory hath rendered our Kingdom safe from all Invasion or suspicion of peril WE THEREFOR willing to reward such laudable a service to Us (as is aforesaid) done and rendered of our special grace and of our certain knowledge and mere motion and also at the humble petition of the said Earl of Nottingham have given granted and by these presents for Us our heirs and Successors DO GIVE and GRANT to our beloved subjects Nicholas Zouche Esquire and Thomas Ware gentleman servants of the aforesaid Earl their heirs and assigns all those our Manors of Donyngton Winterborne Davers alias Winterborne Danvers Winterborne Mayne and Leakehampsted in our Counties of Berks and Wilts or the other of them with all their rights members and appurtenances AND those rents of Assize and our services of our free Tenants in Donynton Winterborne Davers alias Winterborne Danvers, Winterborne Mayne and Leakehampstead in our Counties of Berks or Wilts or in any of them AND all those our rents farms and services of Customary Tenants either by Copy or Court Roll in Donynton Winterborne Davers alias Winterborne Danvers Winterborne Mayne and Leckhampstead aforesaid or in any of them. And all those our perquisites and profits of our Courts of the Manors aforesaid AND all that our Castle of Donyngton with the appurtenances in Donyngton aforesaid in the said our County of Berks and all that our Park of Donynton with the appurtenances and all deer and beasts of chase being in the same Park in the said our County of Berks AND all that meadow called Lord's Meade alias Horsemeade with its appurtenances in Donyngton aforesaid in the said our county of Berks AND all those our two watermills of Donyngton aforesaid with their rights and all their appurtenances set and being in Donyngton aforesaid. . . . . . . '

'. . . . . . LIKEWISE the advowson free donation disposition and right of patronage of the Almshouse or Hospital of Donyngton in the said County of Berks. . . . '

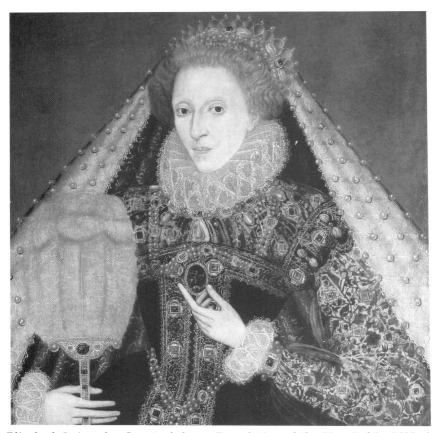

Elizabeth I signed a Grant of the re-Foundation of the Hospital in 1602, in return for which one red rose was to be presented annually to the sovereign by the Lord of the Manor of Donnington.

The grant, though not so expressed in the patent, was apparently subject to a trust in favour of the Earl and Countess and accordingly, by an indenture dated 20th December, 1601 and enrolled in Chancery on the following 7th January, Zouche as the surviving patentee conveyed Donnington to the Earl and Countess for life with the remainder to their son William Howard and the heirs male of his body lawfully begotten and then similarly to their son Charles, and the three sons of the Earl's brother, Sir William Howard, in succession, and finally to the heirs and assigns of the Earl.

Evidently the decayed and ruinous state of the almshouses was a cause of concern to the Earl. In 1601 he appointed a new minister, John Duke, to administer the charity, an appointment which was to last for the next seven years. Also, he sought permission from the Queen to rebuild the hospital, presumably at his own expense.

The Grant of Re-foundation was signed by Elizabeth I on the 25th November, 1602. It stated that the new hospital was to be built on the existing site and called 'Queen Elizabeth's Hospital'. As in the past it was to provide for twelve poor men and their minister. The Statutes and Ordinances were to be made by the Patron and Minister, with the consent of the Archbishop of Canterbury, as to the religion and divine service within the Hospital, and also the salaries of the almsmen.

In return for the Grant a red rose was to be presented annually to the Sovereign. The date arranged for this presentation was 24th June.

'To hold the aforesaid house manor messuages lands tenements and all and singular other things mentioned above of the aforesaid Charles Earl of Nottingham his heirs and assigns as of his manor of Donnington aforesaid in our County of Berks. by a rent of one red rose to be paid annually and faithfully at the feast of the Nativity of St John the Baptist for all rents and services whatsoever'
(Translated from Patent Roll 44 Eliz Part 18 M4
25th November 1602 – Public Record Office)

Although John Duke obviously supervised much of the hospital's administration while the Earl of Nottingham concerned himself with affairs of national importance, some of the illustrious owner's attention was focused upon Donnington during the years that the hospital was being rebuilt.

King James I and his Queen, Anne of Denmark, on whom he had bestowed the manor of Newbury as part of her dowry, decided to visit the town very early in the new reign. In September 1603, the royal couple were the guests of Sir Thomas Dolman, the wealthy clothier who resided at Shaw House, but as there was insufficient accommodation for the Queen's retinue, the Earl placed Donnington Castle at the disposal of the Court. This did not please Lady Russell who, in spite of Queen Elizabeth's grant to the Earl, still considered herself the rightful Keeper of the Castle. She certainly had no intention of being ousted on the occasion of a royal visit.

The displeased lady was in Wales on a visit to her daughter Anne, Lady Herbert, and as soon as the news reached her that workmen were about to enter the castle to make the necessary arrangements for the expected guests, she issued orders that no workmen were to be admitted. She then travelled post haste to Donnington to ensure that her orders were obeyed. When she arrived she was furious to discover that the Earl's servants had made a forced entry. Furthermore, they would not allow her to enter the castle. Momentarily rebuffed the outraged Keeper retreated to Newbury.

The following day Lady Russell and the Mayor of Newbury, accompanied by a band of clothiers all of whom were armed with some sort of weapon, rode to the castle. The cavalcade must have been watched with interest by the villagers and almsmen and provided ample food for gossip for weeks to come. The brave show was of no avail – no admittance was gained at the castle or the lodge (on the site of the present Donnington Castle House) which was the official residence of the Keeper of the Castle.

The redoubtable Lady Russell was not easily defeated. A few days later she personally petitioned the king hoping that he would support her claim. He had been on a short visit to Winchester at the height of the friction but returned to Shaw House in time to hear a first-hand account of the dispute. Wisely, he refused to be drawn into the controversy and referred Lady Russell to the Court of the Star Chamber. Her grievances were heard on May 14th 1606, when she asserted that the castle should have remained under her jurisdiction during her lifetime. Her defence was spirited to say the least; she seized the Earl of Nottingham by his cloak, and even the Lord Chancellor could not stop her tirade of abuse to all who opposed her claim. It was not surprising that she lost her case and that judgement was given in favour of the Earl.

Another episode which must have caused the Earl considerable concern took place in 1614 when his son, William, Lord Howard of Effingham, as heir apparent, bargained and sold the manor and park together with the advowson, donation, and free disposition and rights of patronage of the almshouses, or Hospital of Donnington, to Peter Vanlore of Tylehurst, probably by way of settling a mortgage. Peter Vanlore, having omitted to obtain a licence for the purpose, was pardoned for the offence on 13th May 1616, by which time Lord Howard of Effingham was dead. After the matter had been settled the manor was granted by licence to

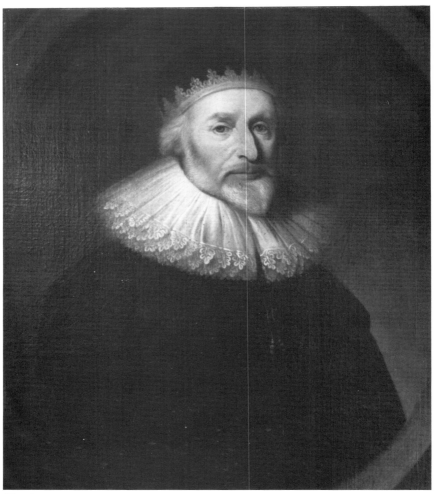

Charles, Baron Howard of Effingham, Earl of Nottingham

his widow, Anne, for her lifetime, then to their daughter Elizabeth and the heirs of her body.

During this period the restoration of the hospital was completed and new rules were drawn up by the Earl of Nottingham and the then minister, Richard James, with the consent of the Archbishop of Canterbury. They are dated 4th March in the 16th year of James I (1619).

Appointment of Men.	1. There shall be for ever a Master and twelve Men; the Earl of Nottingham, his heirs or assigns, to appoint such Master or Almsmen within three months after vacancy, or else the King to appoint.
Not to be Absent without leave.	2. Not to lodge out without the consent of the master; to forfeit 1d. for every night absent, and for every week 6d. to be given to the others; if absent twenty-eight nights to forfeit one quarter's salary to be applied to repairs etc.
No Stranger.	3. No Stranger, Man or Woman, to lodge or harbour in the Hospital. Almsmen harbouring either to lose their Rooms etc.
Good Order.	4. No Drunkard, Common Swearer, Gamester, Tavern Visitor, Brawler, or Fighter, or Notorious Offender, (being warned three times by the Master) be suffered to remain.
Porter.	5. A Porter to be named by the Master for every Quarter of the Year; to keep the keys of the Gate and open and shut them from Lady Day to Michaelmas at six or seven in the morning and eight o'clock at night; and from Michaelmas to Lady Day at seven or eight in the morning and five o'clock at night; and give caution as to fire.
Divine Service.	6. All but the Porter to go to Church on Sundays and Festival Days, and on Mondays, Fridays, and Saturdays, if there is service, in a seemly manner together, and twice a year to receive the sacraments.
Rent.	7. Rents to be received by the Master and disbursed.
Portions.	8. The Master to take yearly 3⅛ Quarters of Wheat, or the price at 6s.8d. per Quarter; and every day take 4d. of cash from Yistely; and each of the men 1⅛ quarters, or the price at 6s.8d. and 2d. daily, by the Week in the Hall of the Hospital and no other place; being the proper proportion.
Provisos.	– Provided, and it shall be lawful to alter Weekly or Quarterly payments; if rents increase or be of more value, to increase stipend in the same proportion.
Accompt Yearly.	9. The Patron to appoint a person to take Accompt in the Hospital yearly, between the feast of St. Michael and the birth of our Lord God, in the

presence of the 12 Men, and give them Notice; and render an open and just and true accompt.

Leasing.
10. No Lease be granted but by consent of the Master and a Majority of the Men, nor unless the accustomed yearly rents or more, be reserved payable half yearly.

Fines, etc.
11. Fines, Woodfalls, and all other casual Income, to be kept as Stock until it amount to £20 for reparations and Extras; and not to be employed without the consent of the Master and the greater part of the Almsmen. And the residue of such casual profits to be distributed by the Master in the same proportions as the annual rents and profits.

Com. Chests.
12. To have two Chests in one of the rooms:-
1 to have 3 locks and Keys of several Wards. – 1 for the Master, 1 for the eldest Almsman, and one for the other Almsmen. In this chest is to be kept the Common Seal, the Charter of Foundation, all Deeds, Leases, etc., and the Ordinances belonging to the Hospital. Also in this Chest, a book in which shall be entered when any Deed or thing is taken out of the Chest; by whom and when returned.

Ledger Books.
The other Chest to have 2 Locks and Keys for 3 Ledger Books. In one of which shall be entered from time to time the names of the Master and Almsmen, the times of their Admission, and their death or removal. In one other Book copies of all Leases, and of all Grants made by the Hospital, or which may be made. And in the third an Inventory of all moveables and gifts of Benefactors and their names. The accompts of the Master, and all other things of any Moment which shall happen.

Part of Minister's Duty.
13. The Master to provide the Chests, etc., and the Books, etc. and to write, or cause to be written, all matters or things concerning the Hospital. To keep the Keys of the Vacant Rooms, and deliver to Almsmen to occupy. Men to pay 2s. 6d. on admission for the benefit of the house. To exact and keepe Accompts, and exhort, and reprove, and inform the Patron.

Repairs.
14. If any Glass be broken, or other decay by wilfulness or neglect in any private room, to be

amended by the Men, or forfeit 2d. per week
until done, and one of the Almsmen to be
appointed by the Master to oversee the works
and reparations, and to give notice of defects that
they may be repaired.

Begging.   15. None to beg, but may receive what is given to the
Hospital in general, or to any one private Alms-
man.

Trade.   16. Almsmen may carry on any handicraft or manual
trade in the Hospital, but not to keep any ale or
victualling house without the license of the
Master.

Sickness.   17. To assist one another in sickness, and Master
may appoint a Brother for that purpose, and pay
him.

Disputes.   18. All disputes to be settled by the Patron and Master of the Hospital (and none other) and the Men
shall not complain to any other; and any that do
otherwise, shall be expelled from the Hospital.

19. The Patron and Master to interpret any doubt or
question concerning the ordinances or Management of the aforesaid Hospital.

NOTTINGHAM

C. CANT.   RICHARD JAMES.

(The above translation of the Rules and Ordinances for the Government
of Donnington Hospital was taken from *The History and Antiquities of
Newbury and its Environs* published 1839)

The new rules seemed designed to ensure the well being of
the hospital, minister and almsmen but the minister, Richard
James, who had been appointed in 1608, flagrantly broke the rules
to his own advantage and that of his relatives. He lived in the
manor house at Iffley and was rarely seen in Donnington. Furthermore, he not only used the income from the manor of Iffley for
his own needs rather than those of the hospital but he leased lands
at Iffley worth £110 a year to his brother-in-law, Humfrey Sutton,
for a fine of £120 and a yearly rent of £12.

To add to these shortcomings he accepted a bribe of £12 from a
fellmonger of Oxford, George Phipps, and admitted him as an
almsman, although in fact, Phipps was reputed to be a wealthy
man worth £1,000. This nomination was not made by the patron;
another breach of the rules.

At this period the hospital was largely occupied by old soldiers who had given good service to their country, but gradually their numbers decreased until there were only two or three actually living in the almshouses.

A sorry state of affairs so soon after the refoundation of the charity but no doubt the hospital was suffering from the division between the patrons and the resident lords of the manor of Donnington.

The first Earl of Nottingham died in 1624 and his heir was Charles, the second son by his first marriage. Charles died without male issue in 1642 and in turn was succeeded by his half brother, who was also named Charles. He was the son of the first Earl's second marriage to Margaret, daughter of the Earl of Murray.

Lady Anne Howard of Effingham, widow of the Earl's eldest son William, retained her interest in the manor of Donnington together with her daughter, Elizabeth, who had married John Mordaunt, Earl of Peterborough, but there were financial difficulties and in the early 1630s it appears that John Chamberlain of Newbury was the owner of Donnington Castle for a brief period. However, in 1632 the manor and castle were purchased by John Packer, lord of the manor of Shellingford in Berkshire, and private Secretary to George Villiers, Duke of Buckingham.

In spite of the changes in ownership of the manor the successive earls retained their right of patronage of the hospital as heirs of the founder. Even before the Peterboroughs relinquished the manor confusion had arisen over the administration as reported in a statement made by George Starkey in June 1634 when proceedings in Chancery were instituted respecting the hospital.

George Starkey deposed that 'he was the receiver of the rents of the manor of Donnington etc. for the late Lord Effingham and that Lady Howard and Lord Peterborough did conceive themselves to have placing of almsmen in the said hospital, and because such as they did present was rejected by Mr James, the minister of the hospital, the hospital was in much decay, and that the almsmen did most, if not all, live abroad.'

This state of affairs was confirmed by John Parsons of Snelsmore, John Northcroft of Newbury, Thomas Knight of Speen, and Henry Smith of Donnington. John Head of Donnington added 'There is not, nor for many years, have been to the knowledge of this deponent either the minister, or any poor men at all inhabiting the hospital.'

Richard James died in 1643 and Humfrey Sutton acted quickly upon his brother-in-law's death. He procured from Charles Howard, 3rd Earl of Nottingham, an election to the hospital, and by some means obtained possession of the Common Seal, although he had not the keys of the muniment chest – apparently only a slight deterrent to so determined a rogue. He demised to his sister for twenty-one years the premises he held at Iffley without fine and at the rent of £50, and 16 acres more (worth £10 yearly) for two fines of £21 each and at a yearly rent of 4d., payable only if demanded, and other lands at Hockmorrow Street in Iffley (worth £24 yearly) at the yearly rent of £6. Perhaps it was as well for the hospital that Sutton died in 1644 and in December of that year the 3rd Earl appointed another minister, Richard Lawrence. Unfortunately he seems to have done little, if anything, to improve the hospital's finances but his appointment came at a difficult time when the country was engaged in civil war and in 1644 Donnington became embroiled in the conflict.

The Civil War Comes to Donnington

In spite of his loyal service to the Duke of Buckingham, one of King Charles I's closest friends, John Packer, the new owner of Donnington, fell from royal favour when he refused to lend money to the king in 1640. Packer joined the ranks of the king's opponents with the result that Charles considered it imprudent to leave Donnington Castle in his hands during the Civil War. The fortress, although small, dominated the roads from London to the West Country, and from Southampton to Oxford, the headquarters of the Royalists. It was, therefore, sequestered by the king and placed under the command of Sir John Boys with orders that it must be held against all opposition, orders which were faithfully obeyed by the gallant commander and his men when the castle was besieged by the Parliamentary forces from 1644 to 1646.

During the autumn of 1645 Sir John decided that the houses in Donnington village must be razed to the ground in order to deprive the Parliamentarians of shelter. He was expecting renewed attacks under the command of Colonel Dalbier who had arrived in Newbury after the successful storming of Basing House. With the other villagers the remaining almsmen, probably only two in number, watched their homes burn until the ruined buildings were incapable of harbouring the enemy.

Severe winter weather must have brought great hardship to the homeless. It also delayed Dalbier's attack but in the early spring the badly damaged castle faced heavy mortar fire but still the brave defenders fought on despite all odds.

By March, 1646, it was apparent that the king's cause was lost. Colonel Dalbier wrote to Sir John Boys advising him to yield soon 'whilst he might be able to give him conditions'. Two messengers were sent to Oxford to receive the king's instructions. They returned with orders to surrender on the best possible conditions that could be obtained.

Subsequently 'the Castellians were to marche awaye to Wallingeforde with bagge and baggage, muskets chargd and primed, mache in Coke, bullate in mouth, drums beatinge and Collurers ffleyinge. Every man taken with him as much amunishion as hee could Carye. As honourable Conditions as Could be given. In fine, thus was Denington Castell surrendered.'

On the 1st April 1646, Donnington was at peace, its castle shattered, its houses and its hospital in ruins. Sir Richard Abberbury would have been heartbroken to see, seemingly, the end of his dreams. But one thing remained intact, his gatehouse, damaged perhaps, but his very own contribution to the building of the castle had withstood the siege, to be a reminder for centuries to come of the brave defence of Donnington Castle.

It now remained for the people of Donnington to rebuild their homes and resume their interrupted work and pastimes under the Commonwealth regime.

The Rebuilding of the Hospital

John Packer must have been dismayed as he gazed upon the devastation caused by the Civil War in Donnington. He is reputed to have rebuilt the old Keeper's lodge with materials from the ruined castle, but he died in 1649 and the major work of restoration to what is now Donnington Castle House, the hospital and the manor in general fell upon his son and heir Robert Packer and a younger son, William Packer.

Although the almsmen were lodged elsewhere, the administration of the hospital's property and finances was a matter of importance. Lawrence, the minister, appears to have been unequal to the task and he disappeared without trace in 1652, leaving the affairs of the hospital in a state of chaos.

The absentee minister was replaced by Walter White by the patron, the 3rd Earl of Nottingham. Although denied the patronage and therefore the right to appoint the ministers it fell to the lot of the Packers to bring order out of chaos at the hospital.

In 1652 Commissioners were appointed to examine the affairs of the charity. They found that the corn rents had not been paid for twenty years, that John Weedon had owned Sulthorpe for twenty years, Roger Brent owned Thropp, John Packer, deceased, and Robert Packer, his son and heir, had been seised of the Manor of Donnington for twenty years, Philip Weston had purchased Bussock in 1650, and that Winterbourne Mayne was owned by various members of the Pocock family.

Time was allowed for enquiries to be made regarding the irregularities which had occurred over the years and the Commissioners met again at Farringdon on the 11th August 1653. They then directed that the hospital should be rebuilt and furnished as before. William Packer was appointed as receiver to collect the arrears of money owing to the hospital and was authorised to receive the current incomes, out of which he was to pay £61. 12s. yearly and the corn money, for the maintenance of the minister and poor men until the rebuilding was completed. The rebuilding was to be carried out within five years.

Improper leases were quashed by the Commissioners and the lessors were ordered to pay the arrears of the difference between the rents reserved and the annual values. Phipps, the almsman who was illegally admitted by Richard James, was removed from the list of almsmen and ordered to pay £40 as reimbursement for the benefits he had received over a period of ten years, a nasty jolt for one who must have thought he had managed to defraud the charity very cleverly.

The new master, Walter White, had to find two sureties for his duly accounting annually for the profits coming into his hands. The Commissioners seemed intent on placing the hospital's finances on a firm and fair basis!

Another matter was raised at the 1652 inquiry – the whereabouts of the chest containing the muniments and ledger books which had disappeared during the time of the burning of the hospital. It was stated that one of three keys had been deposited by the minister and poor men with Humfrey Dolman of Shaw House. Subsequently, Thomas Dolman gave evidence at Speenhamland on the 16th January 1655, that he had seen the grant of Sir Richard Abberbury, and that it was delivered to him with other writings by the Commissioners of 1652. It seems possible, therefore, that Humfrey Dolman not only had the key but the chest itself. Sir Thomas Dolman died in 1697 and it appears that the deeds were redelivered to the hospital where they remained until the disappearance of the then Master, Mr Graham, in the 19th century. Perhaps one day, somewhere, the original grant will be rediscovered!

However, that matter did not concern William Packer who was responsible for seeing that the Commissioner's orders were obeyed, a responsibility which he found irksome at times judging by a letter which is still in existence, dated 11th January 1656. It is addressed:

> This
> for Mr. Walter White Master
> of the Hospital in Donnington
> at his Chambers in the Inner
> Temple, London.

Leave this at the Ancore over agt. St. Dunstan Church London to be remov'd to him with care.

Mr. White.

I have rec[d] yours of the 3rd instant and cannot but wonder that you have not rec: more from me for I have answer'd all that you sent, and if they have miscarried it must be the fault of the carrier of post by whom I sent them. I have rec: intelligence from Oxford that the money is return'd and I do purpose to pay it tomorrow to the party that return'd it from Oxford and concerning this I have writt to Dr. Miller which will produce a speedy payment of you as I have long desired and indeavoured but returnes are both uncertain and deceiptful. I hope there will need no more letters about this. As for your Orchard I shall not meddle with it this yeare because I have not the consent of all. I find it is but a thankeless office to minde the good of others. Richard Almans memory failes him concerning his payment for I paid him but forty foure shillings as I did the other two and so much it comes to at £61.12s. p.ann. in the whole as you may cast it. Thus hoping that these resolve heates agt. me who have not reapt any advantage to myself in this troublesome employment but wholy minded yo[rs] and yo[r] Brethrens' benefit as shall in a short time appeare.

I remain
Your . . . ffriend
William Packer.

Shellingford Hse.
11th. January, 1656.

At the time of this letter William Packer must have been concerned also with the rebuilding of the hospital as four years had elapsed since the 1652 inquiry. It is not certain when the work was completed but an Order of Chancery made on the 12th June 14 Charles II (1662) directed Walter White, the minister, to give notice to the poor men to return to the hospital. This suggests that the hospital was then ready to receive them. If so, the rebuilding had taken ten years instead of the five allotted by the inquiry – a cause of further anxiety to William Packer.

However, the affairs of the hospital were gradually brought under control. New leases were arranged, rents were collected and accounts kept and audited. A lease dated 1670 and still extant is a typical example of the transactions at this period.

'This indenture dated the two and twentieth day of April in the two and twentieth year of the Reign of our Sovereign Lord Charles II by the Grace of God of England, Scotland, France and Ireland King, defender of the faith Anno Dmi 1670 between Walter White Gent. Minister of the Hospital of Queen Elizabeth in Donnington heretofore by Richard Abberbury Knt. begun to be founded by Charles Howard late Duke of Nottingham perfected and consummated and the poor men of the said Hospital of the one parte and Joseph Sawyers of Cholesly in ye County of Berks yeoman of the other pte witnesseth that the said Minister and poor men of the said Hospital as well for and in consideration of the summe of five pounds of good and lawfull money of England to them in hand paid by the said Joseph Sawyer at or before the sealing and delivery hereof as also the surrender up on a bond of twenty years which Ralph Sawyers of Yeftley in the County of Oxon. Gent. had in the premises at the granting hereof but for diverse and other good reasons and considerations them hereunto have in the whole assent, consent and agreement Demised Granted and to farm letten and do by these presents demise grant and to farm lett unto the said Joseph Sawyer his exors heirs ands assignes all that their farme called Denniford Granted and to farm in the .... plan of Yeftley aforesaid together with all the lands meadows and pastures........'

Accounts of 1670 show the receipts and disbursements of the rents and corn rent.

Rec'd The Midsummer Grass money 1670 the summe of eight pounds 15 shilling.	8. 15.	0.
received of John Adams for the Common plot.	10.	0.
received for a heriot.	1. 10.	0.
The totall receipts	10. 15.	0.

Disbustment

Richard Jordan	0. 12.	6.
Daniell White	0. 12.	6.
John Ellots	0. 12.	6.
Francis Spicer	0. 12.	6.

William Manfield	0.	12.	6.
Tho. Smith	0.	12.	6.
Francis Rowland	0.	12.	6.
William Whistler	0.	12.	6.
William Trinity	0.	12.	6.
Tho. Hidin	0.	12.	6.
Widdo Dowman	0.	12.	6.
Richard Moore	0.	12.	6.
Walter White for my owne pay	1.	5.	0.
Paid to the Steward for his fee last Lady Day past.	2.	0.	0.
The total Disburst	10.	15.	0.

Rec'd the Mickelmas Rent 1670 Due for the proffits of the Hospitall of Donnington.

Received for the Grate farme of Yeftley of Mr. Saunders and Mr. Sayer	30.	0.	0.
Received for Hockmore farme	3.	0.	0.
Received for Coppie and freehold rents	10.	3.	4.
Received of Mr. Weston for his Corne rent	1.	4.	9.
Received of Robert Packer Esquire for his corne rent	1.	4.	9.
Received of Peeter Holmes for the acre in the field	0.	6.	0.
Received of Will Whistler for the orchard	0.	6.	0.
Received of Giles Poocock for Corne rent	—	—	
Received of John Poocock for Corne rent	0.	4.	0.
Received of Thomas Sare of Houngerford	0.	6.	8.
The sume is	46.	15.	6.

Disburst for Mich'mas 1670

Paid to Richard Jordan	3.	6.	9.
To William Trinity	3.	6.	9.
To John Elliott	3.	6.	9.

To Daniell White	3.	6.	9.
To Thomas Hidden	3.	6.	9.
To Francis Rowland	3.	6.	9.
To Francis Spicer	3.	6.	9.
To Richard Moore	3.	6.	9.
To Thomas Smith	3.	6.	9.
To Alexander Bromly	3.	6.	9.
To William Whistler	3.	6.	9.
To Henry Manfield	3.	6.	9.
To the Paymaster	6.	13.	6.
The Total disbursem'ts	46.	14.	6.

There is remayning of			
stocke in the Chest this	l.	s.	d.
21th Octob'r 1670	11.	7.	6.

Taken & Audited before the Master & Maior
parte of the Almesmen this 21th Octob'r 1670   per me
William Packer   appoynted auditor.

William Packer had the satisfaction of seeing his work completed in spite of the frustrations and delays which beset him at times. The hospital was rebuilt and its affairs in order before he died in 1679. Soon afterwards the question of the patronage was resolved. The 3rd Earl of Nottingham died without issue in 1681 and the title became extinct. The patronage of the hospital at last passed to the Packer family as lords of the manor of Donnington.

Robert Packer, who had married Temperance Stephens of Little Sodbury in Gloucestershire, also died in 1681 leaving the manors of Donnington and Shellingford in the possession of his wife, as her jointure. A steward, possibly Michael Mallet who, according to Mr Walter Money, was a barrister of some importance, appears to have administered the estates at this time. As it transpired this was a providential arrangement, for John Packer, the son and heir of Robert Packer, outlived his father by only one year leaving his five year old son, Robert, to succeed him. It was as well that during his long minority, Robert's interests were in the hands of his grandmother and a competent steward.

In 1686 Ralph Saunders was appointed as minister by the new patron and the following deeds were executed within the next decade.

This Indenture made the first day of July in the fifth year of the reign
of our Sovreign Lord and Lady William and Mary by the Grace of
God of England Scotland France and Ireland King and Queen
Defender of the Faith and in the year of our Lord God one thousand
six hundred ninety and three between Ralph Saunders Gent. Minister of the Hospital of Queen Elizabeth in Donnington heretofore by
Richard Abberbury Knight begun to be founded and by Charles
Howard, late Earl of Nottingham, deceased, perfected and consummated and the poor men of the said Hospital of the one part and
John White late of Yeftley in the County of Oxon husbandman of the
other part witnesseth that the said Minister and poor men for and in
consideration of the sum of twenty shillings to them in hand paid by
the said John White on the sealing and delivery of these present and
for diver other good and valuable causes and considerations them
hereunto have demised granted and to farme letten and by their
assents do demise grant and to farme lett unto him the said John
White all that their acre of meadow ground commonly called or
known by the name of the Lords Acre lying and being in the
Common meade of Yeftley aforesaid heretofore in the tenure or
occupation of Edward Stubbs or his assignes and also all that their
one acre and a half of meadow ground lying and being in the
common meade of Yeftley aforesaid heretofore in the tenure or
occupation of John Winter or his assignes to have and to hold the
said two acres and a half of meadow ground unto him the said John
White his heirs and assignes for and during the natural lives of him
the said John White, Elizabeth White, the wife of the said John
White and Henry White son of the said John and Elizabeth and the
life of the longer liver of them. Yielding and paying therefore yearly
during the said terme unto the said Minister and poor men and their
successors one pound thirteen shillings and fourpence of lawfull
money of England on the Feast Day of St. John the Baptist at the
manor house at Yeftley without any deduction or defalcation whatsoever for or by reason of any taxes or payments wherewith the
premises hereby demised are or shall be charged by act of Parliament or otherwise during the said term and if it shall happen the
said yearly rent of one pound thirteen shillings and fourpence or
any parte thereof to be behind and unpaid after the said feast in any
yeare during the said term and no sufficient distress to be found on
the said two acres and a half of meadow ground that then and from
thenceforth it shall and may be lawfull to and for the said Minister
and poor men and their successors into the said two acres and a half
of meadow ground to reenter and the same to have again reposess
and enjoy as in their former estate. This indenture or anything
herein contained to the contrary in any wise notwithstanding In

witness whereof to the one part of the Indentures remaining with the said John White the said Minister and poor men have set their Common Seale and to the other part thereof remaining with the said minister and poor men the said John White hath set his hand and seale the day and yeare first above written.

Sgd. John White

Sealed and delivered
in the presence of Tobias Paine
Cha. Fry.'

'This Indenture made the Six and Twentieth Day of March in the Sixth year of Their Majesties reign that now and is in the year of our Lord One Thousand Six Hundred and Ninety Four between Ralph Saunders Gent. Minister of the Hospital of Queen Elizabeth in Donnington heretofore by Richard Abberbury Knight begun to be founded and by Charles Howard, late Earl of Nottingham, deceased, perfected and consummated and the poor men of the same hospital on the one part and Tobias Paine of the city of Oxford Brazier on the other part witnesseth that the said Minister and poor men in consideration of the surrender of the lease for years made of the Lands hereafter mentioned which by mesne assignment is come to the said Tobias Paine and in consideration of a fine of Ten Pounds to them in hand paid by the said Tobias Paine to the said Minister and poor men have with their whole assent consent and agreemᵗ demised granted and confirmed letton and by this present doo demise grant and confirm lett unto the said Tobias Paine all that their parcell of meadow or pasture ground commonly called or known by the name of the Marsh containing by estimateion fifteen acres or thereabouts (be it more or less) situate lying and being in Yeftley in the County of Oxford and alsoe Comon of pasture for three yard lands for all manner of cattle in the fields and comonable places in Yeftley aforesaid (Except and always reserved out of this Demise and grant unto the said Minister and poor men and their successors all and all manner of timber trees now growing or being or what hereafter shall grow or be in or upon the premises or any part thereof with the liberty of ingress egress and regress to fall cut down and carry away the same) To Have and to Hold all and singular the said parcel of meadow or pasture ground and Comon with the appurtances (Except before excepted) unto the said Tobias Paine his executors heirs and assignes from the feast of the Annunciation of the Blessed Virgin Mary last past before the date hereof until the full end and term of the said twenty years from thence next and immediately following fully to be completed and ended, Yielding and paying therefore yearly during the said term unto the said

Minister and poor men and their successors at or in the Common Hall of the said Hospital situated at Donnington aforesaid the sum of three pounds of lawfull money of England on two the most usual feasts or days of payment in the year. . . . . the feast days of St. Michael the Archangel and the Annunciation of the Blessed Virgin Mary by even and equal parts over and above all Taxes and payments be it by Act of Parliament or otherwise howsoever And if it should happen the said yearly rent of Three pounds or any part or parcell thereof to be behind and unpaid by the space of eight and twenty days next after any of the said feasts or days of payment in any year during the said term in which the same ought to be paid and not sufficient dystress to be found in the demised premises that then and from thenceforth it shall and may be lawfull to and for the said Minister and poor men and their successors into the said premises to re-enter and the same to have again to repossess and enjoy as in their former estate This Indenture or anything herein contained to the contrary thereof in any wise not withstanding In witness whereof to the one part of the Indenture remaining with the said Tobias Paine the said Minister and Poor men have set their Common Seal and to the other part thereof remaining with the said Minister and Poor men the said Tobias Paine hath set his hand and seal the day and year full above written.

(Sgd) Tobias Paine.

Tobias Paine's Counterpart 1694.

In 1699, at the age of twenty two, Robert Packer married Mary Winchcombe daughter of Sir Henry Winchcombe of Bucklebury, an event which was to prove another milestone in the history of the hospital.

His grandmother, Temperance Packer, died in 1705, aged eighty years, a remarkable age for that period when the expectation of life was well under the proverbial three score years and ten.

Robert's wife was not so fortunate. She died at the early age of thirty six, a year after she had inherited the Manor of Bucklebury from her elder sister Frances, Lady Bolingbroke who died childless in 1718. The Bucklebury estates were settled, therefore, on Mary's eldest son, Winchcombe Howard Packer.

The parish registers of the church of St Mary, Shaw-cum-Donnington, gives the first reference to the burial of an almsman in 1721 when Mark Rotear of Donnington Almshouse was buried on April 22nd. Thirteen years elapse before another such entry is

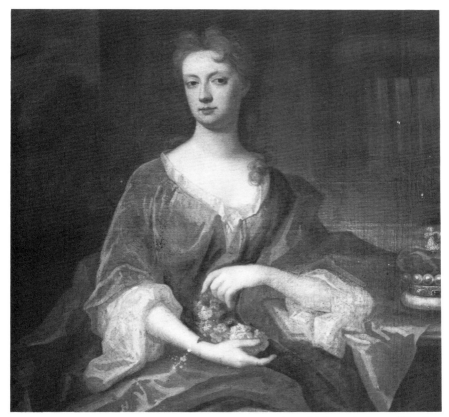

Frances, Lady Bolingbroke. She left the Manor of Bucklebury in her will to her sister Mary Winchcombe, who was married to Robert Packer, Lord of the Manor of Donnington

made, that of William Thatcher who was buried on December 8th 1734. No doubt other elderly men were laid to rest in the village churchyard but the fact that they were almsmen was not recorded by the vicar.

The patron, Robert Packer, died in 1731 leaving the manors of Donnington, Shellingford and Little Sodbury to his son who was, of course, already the lord of the manor at Bucklebury. Two years later the new patron of the hospital, Winchcombe Howard Packer, appointed John Descrambes of Shellingford as the minister of the hospital by the following deed:

'Know all men by these presents that I Winchcombe Howard Packer
of Shellingford in the County of Berks Esquire and Patron of the
Hospital of Queen Elizabeth in Donnington in the County of Berks
aforesaid heretofore by Richard Abberbury Knight begun to be so
founded and by Charles Howard Earl of Nottingham perfected and
consummated Have Given, Granted and Confirmed and by these
presents do Give Grant and Confirm unto John Descrambes of
Shellingford aforesaid Gentleman the office or place of Minister or
Master of the said Hospitall Together with all Lodgings Powers
Authorities Rights Liberties Franchises Revenues Wages Salaries
Stipends Allowances and Profits whatsoever to the said office or
place belonging or appurtaining To have and to hold the said office
or place of Minister or Master of the said Hospitall with all and
Singular the Rights Privileges and Appurtenances whatsoever as
aforesaid to the same belonging or appurtaining unto the said John
Descrambes for and during the term of his natural life according to
the Foundation Statutes and Ordinances of the said Hospital and
not otherwise. In witness whereof the said Winchcombe Howard
Packer have hereunto sett my hand and seal the first day of August
in the seventh year of the Reign of our Sovreign Lord George the
Second King of Great Britain and so forth and in the year of our Lord
One Thousand Seven Hundred and Thirty and Three.
        Sealed and Delivered being
        first July stamp'd in the presence of

John Descrambes held the position until his death in 1738. In
the same year another death was recorded in the Shaw-cum-
Donnington registers, that of Mary Kedwell of Donnington Almshouses. Evidently the wife, or widow, or an almsman, she was
buried on March 6th 1738.

William Law was chosen by the patron to succeed the late
John Descrambes as minister and his deed of appointment is also
extant:

Know all men by these presents that I Winchcombe Howard Packer
Patron of the Hospital of Queen Elizabeth in Donnington in the
County of Berks have freely given granted and confirmed and by
these presents do freely give grant and confirm unto William Law
Gent. the office or place of Minister or Master of the said Hospital
being now void by the death of John Descrambes Gent. Late Minister or Master thereof together with all the Lodgings, Power, Authority, Rights, Liberties, Franchises, Revenues, Wages, Salaries,
Stipends, Allowances, and Profits whatsoever as aforesaid to the
same belonging or appurtaining unto him the said William Law

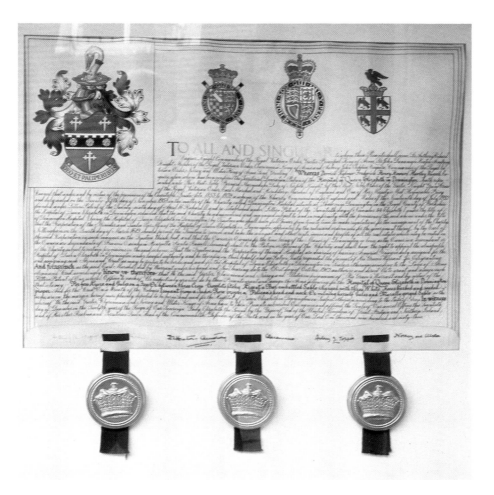

The Grant of Arms of Donnington Hospital

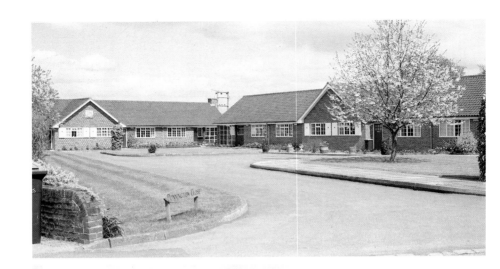

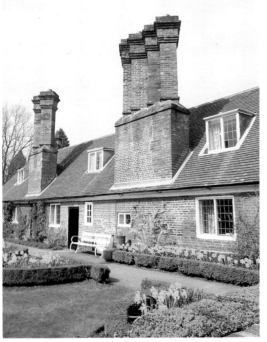

TOP: Donnington Close,
Bucklebury
LEFT: Donnington Hospital
ABOVE RIGHT: Abberbury
Close
RIGHT: Robert Packer, Lord of
the Manor from 1682–1731

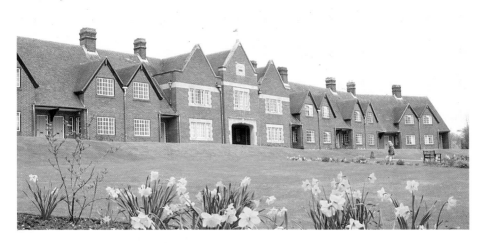

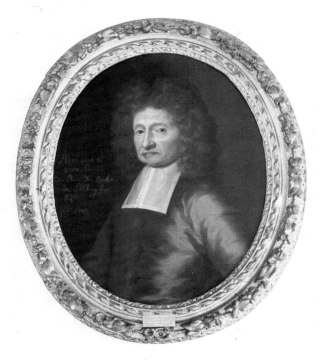

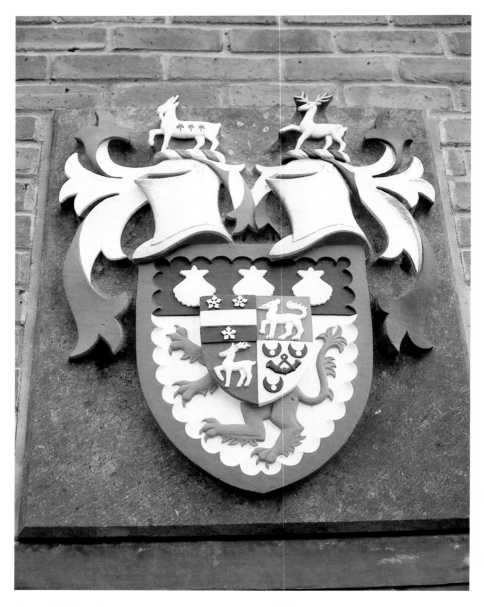

Armorial Bearings at Donnington Close, Bucklebury

from the day of the Date of these presents for and during his Natural life according to the foundation Statutes and ordinances of the said Hospital and not otherwise. In Witness whereof I have hereunto set and affix^d my hand and seal the Twenty Ninth day of October in the twelfth year of the Reign of his Majesty George the Second King of England etc. and in the year of our Lord God One Thousand Seven Hundred and Thirty Eight.

(Sgd) Winchcombe Howard Packer.

On the leaf of the same document the patron made a note of the almsmen:

Richard Poleker	– Sidoll
John Hazell	William Cooper
Thomas Stanbrook	Charles Williams
Gorg. Coox	Mt French
Richard Wintrburn	Zachariah Green for Tobias Davis
Robert Cooks	Geoff. Dane

It is not known for how long William Law remained as minister but it seems likely that on his retirement, or death, he was followed in office by a relative. A lease of 1829 refers to an earlier lease dated 1802 made by a 'Walter Law the then minister'.

In spite of his preoccupation with his various manors, Winchcombe Howard Packer was also Member of Parliament for Berkshire, thus following in his father's footsteps, but he remained a batchelor. On his death in 1746 his estates passed to his younger brother, Henry John Packer, who enjoyed his inheritance for only two months. He died, unmarried, on October 27th 1746. It was tragic that Robert and Mary Packer, having had five sons, left no male heir. Their youngest child and only daughter Elizabeth had married David Hartley the philosopher, and Henry Packer's manors and the patronage of Donnington Hospital passed to his sister's six year old son, Winchcombe Henry Hartley.

On attaining manhood Winchcombe Hartley followed the family tradition and represented Berkshire at Westminster from 1774 to 1790. Ill health dogged his last years and he died of consumption on August 12th 1794, at his London home. He was buried at Bucklebury. His widow, Anne, was left with their seven year old son, Winchcombe Henry Howard Hartley.

Life, and death, went on in the almshouses as in the circles of the patronal family. John Siddal was buried at Shaw on April 4th 1753, Laurence Stephens on October 25th 1767, and two years later, on August 5th, the death of Robert Hellier of Donnington Almshouses was recorded in the parish registers.

Unfortunately, towards the end of the eighteenth century the hospital began to fall into a state of disrepair. No doubt the illness and death of the patron and the minority of his son and heir contributed towards the neglect of the charity but once again the foundation proved resilient enough to weather a stormy passage and emerge as a well ordered house in the early part of the nineteenth century.

Nineteenth Century Revival

The young Winchcombe Henry Howard Hartley matriculated from Merton College, Oxford, on December 9th 1806, when he was eighteen years of age, and later took Holy Orders. He officiated at Bucklebury under the vicar, the Reverend Richard Coxe, but when the incumbent died in 1819 the lord of the manor became the vicar of the parish on his own presentation.

In August, 1809, he had married Elizabeth Watts who not only helped him with his parochial and charitable work but also cared for him during the bouts of ill health which beset him from time to time. They had two children, a son, Winchcombe Henry Howard Hartley, and a daughter, Elizabeth.

The almshouses at Donnington might have been in disrepair at this time but the almsmen were still appointed although many of them, if not all, appear to have lived in their own homes, receiving their pensions and the bounty of their patron. In 1814 Joseph Edge, a tenant of the manor of Bucklebury, was appointed minister.

Fortunately the Reverend Winchcombe Hartley left diaries which contain many references to the hospital and almsmen. These provide information about their day to day lives under his patronage.

1814.
Sunday, 15th. May. I preached my sermon on Rogation week, when I had prayers on Wednesday and full service on Holy Thursday – and a sermon when my poor old men dined with me and walked in my garden.
Wednesday, 7th. December. Wm.* by my appointment with Edge and Wasey visited and reported to me the state of Donnington Hospital.
(*Wm. was William Watts his brother-in-law, and steward of the manor of Bucklebury)

Names	Residence	Age	Recommended by:
1. Jotham Jones	Bath	40	
2. William Body	Tetbury Gloster	60	rec. by Mr. Huntley.
3. Martin Wilkins	Bucklebury	80	
4. Edward Green	do	84	
5. William Ball	do	40	
6. Anthony King	Goodge Street, London	60	
7. Jno Church	Chivelly	64	put in by myself.
8. Thos. Parsons	Bucklebury	77	by do
9. Jeremiah Hope	(as at Frilsham)	70	by me
	do. By		
10. Daniel Clissold	London	52	by Danl*
11. Stephen Johnson	Bucklebury		by me
12. F. Goddard Snr			by me

*N.B. D. Clissold was put in on acct. of past services to my father.
(Notes added later by the Patron record the death of Edward Green on Jan 7th 1817 and William Ball – Nov. 16th. He noted: Cripps elected in the room of W. Ball by me Jno. Andrews elected by me in the room of Edwd. Green deceased.)

1815.
Jan. Mr. Wasey called and took dinner with us. He brought with him a Plan of the repairs of Donnington Almshouses.
Jan. 25th. Our old men dined here.
Nov. 1st. All Saints. Read prayers at Church and entertained twelve old men.

1816.
Jan 25th. Read Divine Service and after entertained the Old Men – some of them vis. Johnson, Amsden, and Old Wigmore were absent.
May 23rd. Ascension Day. Read prayers at Church and according to annual custom entertained twelve old men. 1. Cripps. 2. Amsden. 3. Adams. 4. Fr. Goddard. 5. Jno. Andrews. 6. Steven Johnson. 7. Jeremy Hope. 8. Abram Pendrey. 9. Wait. 10. Clemmonds. 11. Tidbury. 12. –
28th. October. St. Simon & Jude. but poorly and read prayers at Church to ye Old Men who dined here that day.

1817.
Thursday, Jan. 10th. Almsmen promised (1) Pendrey
(2) Lawrence.
List of Old Men to dine here Ash Wednesday.
1. F. Goddard   Carpenter
2. Jno. Andrews
3. Amsden   Freeholder

4. Cripps
5. Adams   (blind)
6. Adams
7. Farmer Parsons resides at Frilsham.
8. Wayte
9. Hope
10. Clemmonds
11. Paulin
12. Tidbury

During the summer of 1817 the Rev. Winchcombe Hartley suffered considerable anxiety over particulars which were issued concerning the sale of the Manor of Wallingford described as 'belonging to his Majesty.' The particulars included 'The Manor of Donnington with all quit-rents, courts, rights, members, and appurtenances – quit-rents and certainty money payable at this court amount annually to 6s.7d. There are about 70 acres of waste within the tithing of Donnington besides several slips of waste by the sides of the roads, some parts of which have been encroached and for which acknowledgements are paid. There is timber on some parts of the waste.' The auction was advertised for 12th August 1817.

As no conveyance of the manor, or any part of it, had been made to the Crown, the Rev. Winchcombe Hartley immediately queried the proposed sale of the Donnington property. Three years of legal controversy followed before he finally submitted and paid £150 for property which he, and others, considered was his own by right of the lordship. By that time he probably thought it less costly to pay the £150 than to continue expensive litigation.

An entry in his diary dated 10th January 1824 throws an interesting sidelight on this episode:

'Recd. a letter from Mr. Bebb claiming a former promise of renewing his lease, which was *conditional* and became void by unexpected events. I was *desirous* of *purchasing certain lands at Donnington put up to auction by the Crown* and Mr. Bebb who likewise desired to become a purchaser promised (and did not) oppose me, on condition of my granting him an extension of his present lease of Donnington Grove. The lands have since been prov'd *to belong to me* as Lord of Donnington Manour.'

However, before that entry was made in 1824 other events

had been recorded in the patron's diary, including one which was the cause of further anxiety:

1818. On Wednesday, April 8th. saw a copy of the Bill filed in Chancery against me and Mr. J. Edge, Minister of Donnington Hospital – directed Mr. Baker (his solicitor) to take advice of able counsel on the subject – how we ought to proceed.

This entry, no doubt, was the result of complaints concerning the condition of the hospital which were made by certain residents of Donnington, in particular by Mr. Francis Parry, a barrister, and author of *The Charitable Donations within the County of Berks*. He wrote, 'The Hospital should be abolished since the minister (or master) and almsmen hold in such contempt the ordinances of the founder, the conditions on which they hold their places – no charity is so egregiously abused from one end of the county to the other.' He added 'that few people, if any, now alive ever recollect an almsman living in it, that it has been almost, if not quite, indictable for a nuisance as a disorderly house.' He does not say who lived in it to cause such nuisance if the almsmen were not there, but it is generally accepted that it was used as a common poor house, and no doubt vagrants found shelter within its walls. For good measure Mr. Parry reported that all the statutes were disobeyed 'except that which directs the master to collect the rents.'

No wonder the patron sought legal advice, but as it happened the Bill was never persisted in as he was already in the process of putting the almshouses in order.

In spite of his own worries he entertained his old men on April 30th 1818, and recorded that 'they dined in comfort and I gave them good counsel.' He must have felt he needed it himself!

The voices of those who criticised the administration of the charity were finally silenced in 1822 when extensive renovations were completed and the *Reading Mercury* reported on the re-opening in their issue of Monday, November 18th, 1822.

'On the 5th. instant the Donnington Hospital, originally founded by Sir Richard Abberbury, Knt. in the reign of King Richard II. and which has lately undergone a thorough repair, was re-opened by the Reverend Winchcombe Henry Howard Hartley, clerk, the patron, who after reading the founder's statutes to the minister, Mr. Joseph Edge, and the almsmen, delivered an address to them on the nature and duties of their situation. After which the patron, minister and almsmen, partook of a plain dinner at the minister's lodgings. The restitution of this long dilapidated Almshouse to a comfortable tenantable condition will, we doubt not, give satisfaction to the lovers and admirers of primitive piety and munificence.'

With his manorial lands and hospital in good order the patron settled down to his parochial duties and the entertainment of his old men, although an oversight on his part surely caused Mr. Belcher unhappiness on one occasion:
May 27th. 1824. Ascension Day. Read prayers to my twelve old men who dined here in comfort. Belcher overlooked.

Another entry shows that the almshouses were in demand:
1824.
July 29th. Sampson, L'lord of the Lower Ship, Woolhampton, applied to me for an almshouse. He may have the first vacancy.

Belcher appears to have been invited on a later occasion according to the following entry:
Nov. 1st. Being All Saints' Day read prayers to my 12 old men and entertained them with a round of beef, pudding, and ale after Church.
Present Old Men.
 1. Thos Cripps   Scotland*
 2. Paulin
 3. Clemmonds
 4. Belcher
 5. Knott   Scotland*
 6. Ts. White   Briff Lane.
 7. Edward Wigmore   Lower Common.
 8. Snell
 9. Fr. Smith
10. Jno Norris
11. F. Cooper
12. Osgood
13. Henry Head
14. Thomas Adams   Slade.
The affectionate thanks and good wishes of the poor souls was truly delightful. Mr. Saxty and I sat and convers^d cheerfully with

them. Blessed be God for making me an humble instrument of God's to such poor souls.
(*Scotland in Bucklebury.)

The number of twelve seems to have been exceeded on the above occasion and it is obvious from the addresses that some almsmen were still living out of the hospital. An entry on November 30th records 'despatch letters to Mr. Baker and Edge to admit an almsman. The houses are full.'

In an entry of early February, 1825, the names of sixteen almsmen were recorded, again with some home addresses, but change was at hand:

1825.
Thursday, February 24th.
Saint Matthias Day. – Sent a letter direct^d to Mr. Baker to summon Mr. Edge and the non resid^c at D. Hosp to reside or resign by Lady Day.

Mr Sampson of the Lower Ship, Woolhampton, soon received good news in answer to his application for an almshouse, but as later entries show (April 8th & Oct. 14th) he changed his mind!

1825.
23rd March. Wrote to Samson app^{ting} him to the vacant almshouse (late Dennis decd.) and to Edge an order for his admission on his application. (Another entry on the same day explains the presence of female occupants in the Hospital.)
23rd. *D. Hospital.* In cases of almsmen having their wife or other stay^d female relative to reside with them it must be understood to be a special indulgence – and specified – and ye widow must quit the tenement at their decease. All goods belonging to the almsmen go into the common treasury at their decease. No young woman or children to be allowed to reside in the hospital.
– and as an afterthought on the part of the Patron –
March 25th. No woman to take in washing.
April 7th. We all rode over to Donnington Castle where we enjoyed ourselves looking about, and refreshed ourselves. Visited Donnington Hospital which is very tidy and clean in general but on visiting Dibley's, and the tenement occupied by Dennis's widow I observed the walls smoky and the place slovenly, and Dibley's wife was very impertinent.
April 8th. Saw Mr. Sampson of Woolh^{ton} and settled partly for him

to have the refusal of the next vacant almshouse as he cannot leave his Inn at Woolhampton until Michaelmas next 1825 – and then I can fill up Dennis's.

Oct. 14th. Sampson Woolh[ton] declines the almshouse.

Present members of Donnington Hospital.

1. Steele	7. Ilsley
2. Ralph Head	8. Boseley
3. Le Roi	9. Vact. by Church deceased
4. Dibley	10. Vact. by Dennis's decease
5. Vince	11. annexed to the Minister's place
6. Elms	12. Daniel Wheeler

The renovated almshouses were in demand as soon as any became empty and the Patron noted the names of some applicants in his diary:

1825.

October 18th. Mr. Lockett Donn[ton] – A Donnington inhabitant recommended Mr. Best and Colonel Head.
Mr. Pocock of Langley applied.
Mr. Parsons and Wm Adams, timber feller, applied.

October 26th. Mr. Money, Donnington, petitions for an old man nam[d] Hains.

Just a year later on October 26th 1826, a sad message awaited the vicar when he entered his house after taking the service at Bucklebury church. 'On return home recd. tidings of Mr. Joseph Edge's decease – formerly my tenant and Master of Donnington's Almshouses – an application from Mr. Wasey on the subject.'

1826.

October 27th. Our Manorial Court was held. Dr Williams, his daughter and two of his foreign pupils din'd with us and Mr. Hemus (his curate) and his wife – we were all very comfortable and united. Signified my intention of appointing MR. NALDER, Master of Donnington Hospital, to Mr. Baker who highly approv[d] it.

Dec. 14th. Rose well and in good spirits. Appointed Charles Milsom, who is 66 years of age, has brought up 10 children and formerly kept Stanford Dingley mill for 30 years, to the vacant almshouse at Donnington (No. 5)

Charles Milsom was destined to enjoy his new home for only five months. He died the following May and was buried in Stanford Dingley churchyard. The word 'Donnington' was inserted by the entry of his burial in the Stanford Dingley registers. Other almsmen may have been buried in their former parishes thus providing another reason for the small number of almsmen's deaths recorded in the registers of Shaw-cum-Donnington, and those of their wives or other 'stay'd female relatives'.

Only two are recorded for the first half of the nineteenth century: John Skinner, almshouse Donnington, aged 73 years, buried on Jan: 13th. 1828, by Thomas Best, curate, and Sarah Churchill, Donnington almshouse, aged 94 years, buried on April 6th, 1841, by S. Slocock, Vicar.

There appears to have been another application for the mastership of the hospital after the death of Mr. Joseph Edge, according to an entry in the patron's diary dated February 10th 1827. 'Look'd in on Hedges who spoke very properly on my refusal to appoint him master of Donnington Hosp. on the late vacancy. His wife expressed her hope that on some future opportunity I might think on them to which I expressed my inclination to do so.'

A hope that was never realised. Richard Nalder continued in office until 1865, long after the Reverend Winchcombe Hartley had died. Undoubtedly one of the most caring patrons which the hospital had enjoyed to date, Winchcombe Henry Howard Hartley died on September 9th 1832, at the early age of forty five. Not only had he rebuilt the hospital but he had shown personal concern for the welfare of its inmates. They had cause to be grateful to him. The *Reading Mercury* printed the following account of his funeral:

'On Wednesday last the remains of the Rev. W. H. H. Hartley were consigned to the family vault in the church of Bucklebury. The funeral was conducted with that solemnity and propriety which became the rank and situation which he had held in society: the pall was supported by six of the neighbouring clergy: he was followed by his nearest and dearest relations, his numerous tenantry, the twelve aged men, the objects of his bounty, and the children of his school.

The whole population of his extensive parish assembled in crowds to witness the last impressive ceremony over the remains of their beloved pastor, and we may add that more heartfelt and general grief has rarely been more exhibited on such an occasion.'

The twelve almsmen of Donnington had lost a good friend and patron.

Victorian Donnington

The Reverend Winchcombe H. H. Hartley left his estates to his only son, another Winchcombe Henry Howard Hartley, who married Miss Emily Bidenham. His sister, Elizabeth Hartley, married Count Demetrius de Palatiano and her children later became involved with the affairs of Donnington Hospital.

Soon after the young Mr. Hartley came into his inheritance the family home at Bucklebury, a fine old Tudor mansion which had been extensively damaged by fire in 1830, was partially demolished. He found refuge in another of his houses, Lyegrove in Old Sodbury, Gloucestershire, but came to Bucklebury and Donnington from time to time and honoured his obligations as patron of the hospital.

In 1836 in accordance with the Letters Patent issued by Queen Elizabeth I to Charles, Earl of Nottingham, and the authority granted to his heirs and assigns, the patron and the minister, with the consent of the then Archbishop of Canterbury, asserted their right to frame two amended statutes which they considered necessary 'from the change of times and other circumstances.'

'The First disciplinary – imposing a fine of 3s.6d. for each night an almsman absented himself from the hospital without the consent of the master.

The Second financial – providing that Fines of Release, and on admittance to copyhold estates, woodfalls, and all other casual and uncertain profits belonging to the hospital, should be received by the master and kept as stock until it amounted to £100 which sum should be preserved for reparations by the master with the consent of the patron in writing, and that residue of the casual profits should be divided and distributed by the master in the proportions in which the yearly issues and profits are divided namely, quarterly, monthly, or weekly. It was also ordained that upon the death of the master, two-fourteenths parts of the casual profits due

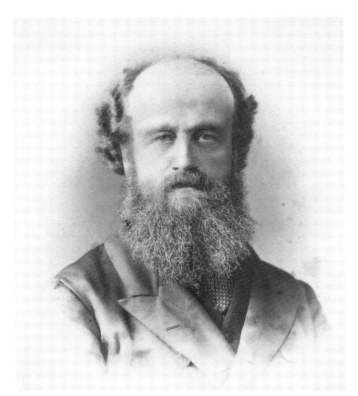

Colonel Winchcombe Henry Howard Hartley, who was Lord of the Manor of Donnington and Patron from 1832–1881

at the time of his death should be deemed part of his personal estate, and paid accordingly, and upon the death of any almsman one-fourteenth part in like manner.

In 1837 a report was issued by the Commissioners of Inquiry concerning charities. They inspected the hospital as much dissatisfaction was expressed on the part of some of the almsmen but the Commissioners satisfied themselves that the complaints were without the slightest foundation. In fact they found the hospital in excellent repair. There were twelve almsmen residing in the hospital, and Thomas Nalder was still the minister. The almsmen were all over sixty years of age and all had been admitted within the last thirteen years. Four were in good employment, two were occasionally employed, and two owned property. Of the two acres once assigned to the almshouses only half an acre remained and this was used as a garden by the almsmen. A quarter of an acre had been taken in 1771 by the trustees of the Newbury and Chilton Turnpike Road, and the remaining acre and a quarter was exchanged in 1776 under an enclosure act for a like quantity of land at Speen.

The Commissioners were concerned with the income of the charity and the uneven distribution of casual profits to the almsmen. They stated that 'the only inconvenience that arises from the practice of letting the property on leases for lives is the uncertain amount of the annual receipt of fines e.g. in 1833 and 1834 only £120 was receive as casual profits but in 1835 and 1836 they amounted to £1,336. 13s. 0d.' The commissioners added that 'as the minister was directed by the statutes to divide quarterly, monthly, or weekly, the casual profits as they are received, the effect is the almsmen, who with scarcely a single exception are improvident, spend in waste all they receive in the good years. It appears to us that their evil way may best be remedied by establishing a reserve fund.'

The matter was still unsettled in 1848. According to the report of the Charity Commissioners issued at the beginning of the twentieth century the Attorney General filed an Information in November 1848 at the relation of Mr. John Hughes who resided at Donnington Priory 'against the minister and twelve poor men, with a view to the amendment of the system of casual profits, which had to a trivial extent been remedied by the statutes of 1836. In the following May the Information was amended for the purpose of raising questions as to the right of patronage, and the improvidence of certain leases. Before this information came for hearing, a second Information was filed, on June 1851, nominally by the Attorney-General at the relation of Edward William Bunny, a clerk in the office of a firm of solicitors, and eight of the almsmen, against Henry Walsh, to whom it was alleged an improvident lease had been granted, the minister and twelve poor men, and four of the almsmen, who had declined to join as plaintiffs. This second Information, it appears, was filed behind the back of the Attorney-General, who repudiated it, and shortly afterwards the court directed all proceedings to be stayed, so that the relators should pay the costs, which amounted to £466.14s.2d.'

So ended one episode in the administrative affairs of the

hospital. Four years later, on the 27th April 1852, a decretal order was made in the first Information by the Master of the Rolls which set out the property belonging to the charity, and ordered that certain leases for twenty one years, which were renewable on the payment of a fine every seven years, of lands containing 182 acres in Iffley should, with one exception, be surrendered, and in lieu thereof leases for forty years should be granted at rents amounting to not less than £280 a year, without any fine. The lease of Henry Walsh was one of those so surrendered and regranted under the forty years' scheme:

'This Indenture made the Twenty fifth day of October one thousand eight hundred and fifty two between THE MINISTER AND POOR MEN of the Hospital of Queen Elizabeth at Donning-ton in times past by Richard Abberbury Knight begun to be founded and by Charles Howard late Earl of Nottingham perfected and consummated (The said Minister and Poor Men being a Body Corporate by virtue of Letters Patent under the Great Seal dated at Westminster the twentieth day of November in the forty fourth year of the reign of Queen Elizabeth) of the one part and Henry Walsh of the City of Oxford Gentleman of the other part Wit-nesseth that in obedience to a Decree of the High Court of Chan-cery dated the twenty seventh day of April one thousand eight hundred and fifty two and made in a cause there then depending between Her Majesty's Attorney General at the Relation of John Hughes Informant and the said Minister and Poor Men of the said Hospital also Thomas Nalder the Minister and Winchcombe Henry Howard Hartley (the Patron) and His Grace the Right Reverend the Archbishop of Canterbury (the Visitor) of the said Hospital as Defendants and in consideration of the surrender of an Indenture of lease dated the thirty first day of October one thousand eight hundred and forty two and made between the said Thomas Nalder Minister and the Poor Men of the said Hospital of the one part and the said Henry Walsh of the other part THEY the said Minister and Poor Men HAVE demised leased set and to farm letten and by these presents in their corporate right and capacity to demise lease set and to farm let unto the said Henry Walsh ALL THAT the Farm, called the COURT PLACE of Yeftley in the County of Oxford AND all the Lands Meadows and Pastures closes Inclosures commons woods underwoods fishings waters ponds brooks parks ways and all other easements and commodities to the same Farm appertaining and belonging AND Also all that parcel of ground called Aldermanbury otherwise Little Kidney with the appurtenances in the County of Berks AND ALSO that piece or parcel of ground called GROVE Close containing by admeasurement Five acres and eighteen perches being numbered 168 on the Plan annexed to the Award of Henry Dixon the Commissioner appointed in and by an Act of Parliament passed in the fifty fifth year of the Reign of his late Majesty King George the third intituled "An Act for Inclosing lands in the Township or Liberty of Yeftley otherwise Iffley within the Manor and Parish of Iffley otherwise Yeftley in the County of Oxford bearing date the ninth day of January one thousand and eight hundred and thirty AND ALSO one other piece or parcel of Land being part of Upper Grove Close containing by estimation four acres two roods and nineteen perches being numbered 170 on the said Plan AND ALSO one other piece or parcel of Land being part of Wheat Close containing two roods and twenty two perches being numbered 165 on the said Plan All which said three last mentioned pieces or parcels of land were parts of a piece or parcel of Land formerly described as ALL THAT parcel of ground commonly called Yeftley Grove heretofore being Wood Ground containing by estimation sixteen acres situate lying and being in the parish of Yeftley in the County of Oxford formerly in the occupation of Joseph Sayer and since of Sarah Coles deceased being parcel of or belonging to the Manor called the Court Place of Yeftley aforesaid And all the underwood thereupon growing or being and all profits and commodities thereunto belonging (Except and always reserved unto the said Minister and Poor Men and their successors All that meadow or Pasture commonly called or known by the name of the Marsh containing by estimation fifteen acres or thereabouts (be the same more or less) lying and being in Yeftley aforesaid AND also except all and all manner of Timber trees now growing or being or which shall hereafter grow or be in or upon the said premises or any part thereof with free liberty or ingress egress and regress to and for the said Minister and Poor Men and their successors and their Agents Servants and Workmen to fell cut down and carry away the same at their will and pleasure) All which Farm and hereditaments hereby demised are now in the tenure or occupation of the said Henry Walsh or of his undertenants and the same are known as the Court

Place or Manor Farm of Iffley and Iffley Grove the later intermixed
with the court Place or Manor Farm aforesaid And the said Farm
hereditaments and premises so intended to be hereby demised do
contain in the whole one hundred and forty two acres or thereabouts and are delineated in the Plan drawn in the Margin of these
presents and the particulars thereof are comprised and set forth in
the Schedule hereto opposite the said Plan TO HAVE and TO
HOLD the said Farmlands and all and singular other the premises
hereby demised or intended so to be (except as before excepted)
unto the said Henry Walsh his executors administrators and
assigns from the twenty-fifth day of March one thousand eight
hundred and fifty two for and during and unto the full end and
term of FORTY YEARS from thence next ensuing and fully to be
complete and ended YIELDING AND PAYING thereof yearly and
every year during the same term unto the said Minister and Poor
Men and their successors at or in the Common Hall of the said
Hospital situate and being at Donnington aforesaid the rent or
sum of TWO HUNDRED POUNDS of good and lawful money of
Great Britain on the twenty fifth day of March and the twenty
ninth day of September in every year by equal and even portions
AND ALSO yielding and paying by like equal portions on the
several days aforesaid the additional yearly rent or sum of Fifty
Pounds of like lawful money for every acre and so in proportion for
any greater or less quantity than an acre of the Meadow or Pasture
ground hereby demised which at any time during the continuance
of this demise shall be ploughed dug broken up or converted into
tillage or garden ground without the license and consent of the
said Minister and Poor Men for that purpose first had and obtained
in writing under their Common Seal and to continue and be paid
and payable during the residue of the said term which shall be then
to come and unexpired AND the said Henry Walsh for himself
his heirs executors administrators and assigns doth hereby covenant grant declare and agree to and with the said Minister and Poor
Men and their successors by these presents in manner following
(that is to say) that he the said Henry Walsh his heirs executors
administrators or assigns shall and will from time to time and at all
times hereafter during the continuance of this demise well and
truly pay or cause to be paid unto the said Minister and Poor Men
and their successors the aforesaid yearly rent or sum of Two
hundred pounds And also the additional rent (in case the same

additional rent shall become due and payable) on the days and times and in the proportions herein before mentioned and appointed for payment thereof without any deduction or abatement thereout or out of any part thereof for or on account whatsoever And also bear pay and discharge all and all manner of taxes charges rates tithe rent charges (if any) assessments or impositions whatsoever which shall or may at any time during the continuance of this demise be rated taxed charged assessed or imposed on the said demised premises or any part thereof by authority of Parliament or otherwise howsoever (The property tax in respect of the said hereby reserved Rent only excepted) And also shall and will at all times during the continuance of this demise well and sufficiently uphold sustain maintain paint pave scour amend and keep as well the Messuage or Tenement Barns stables outhouses and buildings as also all the Gates stiles rails posts pales walls hedges ditches mounds bounds and fences and all and singular other the premises hereby demised in and by and with all and all manner of needful and necessary reparations and amendments whatsoever when where and as often as need or occasion shall be or require upon having sufficient rough timber (if it is to be found on the said demised premises) allowed to him for that purpose And the said Messuage or Tenement Barns stables outhouses and buildings and all and singular other the premises hereby demised being in all things so well and sufficiently repaired upheld supported sustained maintained painted glazed scoured cleaned amended and kept in repair at the end or other sooner determination of the term hereby granted shall and will peaceably and quietly leave surrender and yield up to the said Minister and Poor Men or their successors AND FURTHER that he the said Henry Walsh his executors administrators or assigns shall not or will at any time during the continuance of the term hereby granted plough dig break up or convert into tillage or garden ground any of the Meadow or Pasture land hereby demised without the consent in writing of the same Minister and Poor Men or their successors for that purpose first had and obtained under their Common Seal nor shall nor will at any time during the continuance of this demise manage use or occupy all or any part of the said demised premises contrary to the Known and most approved principles of good husbandry in or near Yeftley aforesaid PROVIDED ALWAYS and these presents are upon these conditions nevertheless that it shall happen that the said yearly rent of Two hundred pounds or the said Additional rent in case the same additional rent shall become due or either of the said rents or any part thereof respectively shall be behind and unpaid for the space of twenty one days next over or after any of the said days of payments whereon the same ought to be paid as aforesaid being lawfully demanded and no sufficient distress be had or found on the said premises whereby to satisfy the same or if the said Henry Walsh his executors administrators or assigns shall at any time or times dig plough break up or convert into tillage or garden ground any of the said Meadow or pasture ground hereby demised or if the said Messuage or Tenement shall become ruinous or shall not be repaired and at all times kept in repair agreeably to the Covenant for that purpose hereinbefore contained that then and in any or either of the said cases it shall be lawful for the said Minister and Poor Men or their successors at any time into and upon the said demised premises or into and any part thereof in the name of the whole wholly to re-enter and the same to have again retain and repossess and enjoy as in their first and former estate and the said Henry Walsh his executors administrators and assigns from there utterly expel put out and amove this Indenture or anything hereinbefore contained to the Contrary thereof in anywise notwithstanding IN WITNESS whereof to the one part of this Indenture remaining with the said Henry Walsh the said Minister and Poor Men have affixed their Common Seal and to the other part remaining with the said Minister and Poor Men the said Henry Walsh hath set his hand and Seal the day and year first above written.'

The attached schedule shows that the area of land involved amounted to 142 acres 3 roods 30 perches. As Henry Walsh signed the new indenture he must have reflected upon the signing of the original lease and the trouble it had caused.

In addition to the renewal of leases on the forty years basis the Commissioners ordered, also, that all leases for three lives, and those for ninety nine years determinable of three lives, should be permitted to expire, and thereupon the premises should be let either at rack-rents for terms not exceeding twenty one years or on building leases for ninety nine years. Certainly this was a more profitable proposition than a three lives lease made in 1823 between the minister and poor men and William Blea, on behalf of Thomas Yearly, aged 54 years, Charles Blea, aged 8 years, and Henry Blea, aged 7 years, upon a fine of £28 paid on the signing of the Indenture and a yearly rent of one shilling payable 'during the lives and life of the longest liver of them'. This lease referred to a cottage and garden in Iffley.

An example of a lease for ninety nine years determinable of three lives was made in 1829 between the minister, Thomas Nalder, and the poor men, and Charles Cripps of Iffley. After an initial fine of £140 a yearly rent of £1.1s.9d. was to be paid for certain land in Iffley 'for and during and unto the full end and term of Ninety Nine years from thence next ensuing and fully to be complete and ended (If the said Charles Cripps party hereto now of the age of thirty three years or thereabouts Charles Cripps son of the said Charles Cripps (party hereto) now of the age of Five years or thereabouts and Ann Cripps daughter of the said Charles Cripps (party hereto) now of the age of Six years or thereabouts or any or either of them shall so long happen to live)' A somewhat optimistic view as even the youngest of the three was unlikely to live for ninety nine years from the date of signing but, at the same time, it would have been possible for one, or all of them, to have enjoyed possession of the land for many years at an extremely low rent.

As such leases lapsed in the years that followed and new ones were granted on terms more compatible with the prosperity of the latter years of the nineteenth century, the income of the charity steadily increased.

Unfortunately the smooth running of the hospital was disrupted by the behaviour of Charles Graham who was appointed minister in 1865 in succession to the long serving Thomas Nalder. Mr Graham, a solicitor of Newbury had appeared to be an extremely suitable candidate for a position of trust. However, it became apparent that the appointment had been a mistake. Graham was a non-resident minister who did little for the hospital, especially on the accounting side. When he finally absconded there was no record of the £220 received from the sale of land at Cowley which had been in the hands of his father who was solicitor to the charity.

In 1877 George Henry Beckhuson, Mr Graham's clerk, became the minister. During his period of office the roof of the hospital was renewed at a cost of three hundred pounds.

It is interesting to note that in a lease granted by Mr. Beckhuson the title of the lessor was simplified and, after so many centuries, the names of Sir Richard Abberbury and the Earl of Nottingham were deleted from the transaction:

'This Indenture made the twenty eighth day of January in the year of our Lord one thousand eight hundred and eighty one Between George Henry Beckhuson gentleman, the Minister of the Hospital of Queen Elizabeth in Donnington in the County of Berks, and the Poor Men of the said Hospital on the one part and Charles Lingham of Iffley in the County of Oxford Esquire of the other part. . . . . .'

This lease must have been one of the last to be made by Mr Beckhuson as his term of office ended during the year in which it was granted and the Patron appointed George J. Watts, a young man of twenty two, as the new Minister. So youthful a man could look forward to a long time in office and, in fact, Mr. Watts held the position until 1932, but the patronage was to change almost immediately.

Colonel Winchcombe Henry Howard Hartley died at his Gloucestershire home on October 31st 1881. He had no children to succeed him and his estates passed to his four nieces, the daughters of his sister Elizabeth, the late Comtesse de Palatiano.

Changes in
Administration

Of the four new patronesses, Elizabeth, Comtesse de Palatiano, Mrs Nina Katherine Webley-Parry, Mrs Olivia Acreman-White, and Mrs Frances Oxenham Henrietta Santa Russell, only Mrs Webley-Parry resided in the neighbourhood, at Bucklebury, and she took a great personal interest in the welfare of the hospital. In 1906 the estates were divided and Elizabeth, Comtesse de Palatiano became Lady of the Manor of Donnington and consequently the patroness of the charitable foundation, but in the intervening years many people busied themselves with the affairs of Donnington almshouses.

Under the new minister the benefits of the increased revenues received from the renewed leases and from the sale of land in Iffley to the Wycombe railway began to be felt, and the stipends of the almsmen were increased from just over ten shillings a week in 1881 to twenty one shillings a week ten years later.

At this time, 1891, Mr Watts purchased a piece of land adjoining the hospital for the erection of a minister's house. It was built, rather mistakenly perhaps, under the headings of 'repairs' and 'materials' in the official accounts, and without the consent of the patronesses and the Charity Commissioners. However, the transaction was given official recognition and the Bridge House as it is called remains the home of the minister to this day.

In 1894 changes occurred in the administration of the charity as the result of information placed before the Charity Commissioners by Colonel Sir Howard Vincent, CB, MP, who lived at Donnington Holt. He considered that the revenues had increased by a hundredfold over the centuries but the number of recipients had remained the same since the day when Sir Richard Abberbury nominated twelve poor men to be the object of his charity. In consequence of his complaint the Commissioners appointed Mr Selby-Biggs, one of the assistant commissioners to hold a local inquiry. It took place in the National Schoolroom of Shaw-cum-

Donnington at 5 p.m. on Wednesday, December 19th 1894.

In his report Colonel Vincent stated the object of the inquiry:

'It is to be hoped that with a view to making the Inquiry both thorough and successful, and to the enlistment of the sympathies of the patroness and all concerned, in attaining the object in view, namely, the greater benefiting of the poor, and especially in the Parish of Donnington, no personal charges or allegations may be made. Doubtless a charity in existence for over five centuries has been attended in the course of years by grave irregularities, and that serious mistakes have been made in its administration. But little or nothing is to be gained by entering into them in detail, or raising hostility with respect to the past. Nor is it sought in any material way to interfere with existing rights or interests. The future is alone to be aimed at.'

The history, conditions and revenues of the charity were fully discussed and the report included a paragraph on the 'Benefits now enjoyed by the Almsmen'.

'At the present time each of the almsmen is receiving 23s.6d. a week in cash, and Quarters. Of the 12 men who are there, ten came from Bucklebury and only two from Donnington. They have a sitting room on the ground floor, and a bedroom over, approached by a steep staircase. The lavatory accommodation is some distance away in the garden. Each of the 12 doors look out on to a small and dreary gravelled courtyard. Most of the old men apparently have their wife or some female relative or attendant to look after them, and a nurse has also, and wisely, been appointed for the infirm.'

The payment of 23s.6d. a week in addition to living accommodation was stated by the Colonel to be out of all proportion to the agricultural wages paid 'to able bodied men having young and too numerous families to support and rent to pay, averaging only from 12s. to 14s. a week – it would seem that a pension of 10s.0d. per week with free furnished quarters, light and fuel, with messing at a fixed charge would be a liberal allowance for future almsmen, whose number might in such case be more than doubled. Indeed I find that in the numerous Almshouses founded by worthy citizens of Newbury in bygone ages, 6s. a week inclusive, or 5s. a week with an allowance of fuel and clothing is usual.'

That part of the Colonel's report must have been extremely unpopular with the almsmen although they probably agreed with his suggestion that some of the surplus revenue should be spent on improving the almshouses; for example, the installation of gas, or even electricity as water power was near at hand, and the general modernisation of the living quarters. He suggested, also, that money should be paid out in pensions to worthy aged poor of Donnington and the Friendly Societies then operating in the parish. He stressed that due to the founder's original statutes the poor of Donnington should be the major beneficiaries of the charity.

Colonel Sir Howard Vincent paid sincere tribute to the work of Mrs Webley-Parry and stated that she was a lady of great administrative capacity who took much interest in the charity.

The outcome of the inquiry resulted in the preparation of a new scheme by the Commissioners which was sealed on the 29th August 1896.

This Scheme directed that the freehold hereditaments belonging to the charity were to remain vested in the Corporation of the Minister and twelve poor men of the Hospital of Queen Elizabeth in Donnington, but the Corporation was to permit the trustees to receive the rents of the estates and manage and use them, and the personal estate of the Corporation, in such manner as the trustees in their discretion thought best. For that purpose the Corporation was to make such deeds, leases, and other instruments, as the trustees required, and the trustees might use the name of the Corporation in bringing or defending actions. All deeds to which the common seal (which was to be kept by the clerk of the trustees) was affixed were to be signed by two at least of the trustees.

The patronage and right of appointment of the minister, almspeople, and pensioners was vested in the owner or owners of the manor and castle of Donnington upon whose default to appoint within three calendar months, unless the Charity Commissioners consented to the extension of that period, the trustees might appoint.

The trustees were at first to be eight in number and consisted of the rector of Shaw-cum-Donnington, ex-officio, and seven representatives to be appointed, three by the patron or patrons, one by the Archbishop of Canterbury, one by the Berkshire County Council, one by the Oxfordshire County Council, and (but only for a period of 8 years from the date of the scheme) one by the

Minister and twelve poor men of the hospital. The nominations of the patron were to be subject to the approval of the Charity Commissioners and a provision was made that in the event of the trustees acquiring the patronage, there would no longer be representatives of the patrons, but in their places, representatives of the parish councils of Shaw-cum-Donnington, Bucklebury, and Iffley, Cowley and Littlemore, as the Charity Commissioners might direct. The representatives of the patrons and the Archbishop of Canterbury were to hold office for seven years, and all others for four years.

Clauses were included as to the meetings and the management of the business of the Trustees who were empowered to appoint proper officers at salaries approved by the Charity Commissioners and provision was made for the repairs, insurance, and management expenses, and the minister's salary and expenses, in addition to the use, free of rent, rates and taxes of the house occupied by him, and the use (free as aforesaid) of his then office in Iffley and his office in the almshouse (unless required for other purpose) with allowances for light and fuel. His salary was fixed at £156 a year with out of pocket expenses when travelling to Iffley on business of the charity.

The Minister's duties were stated as:

a. To manage the estates under the direction of the trustees.
b. To collect all rents and periodical payments and pay them into the trustees' banking account, retaining such cash balances as the trustees thought necessary for minor and current expenses.
c. To pay all allowances to almspeople and pensions and other benefactions.
d. To notify all vacancies among almspeople and pensioners to the clerk.
e. To supervise the discipline of the Hospital and to enforce all rules and regulations made in accordance with the Scheme.

The then steward of the manor of Iffley was to receive the same salary as before and he was to act as clerk and solicitor to the trustees at an inclusive salary of £100. This was to include the preparation of legal instruments but out of pocket expenses for stamps, counsel's fees, agent's charges and travelling expenses were to be paid in addition as were charges for legal proceedings on behalf of the charity when approved by the Commissioners. The rights of the existing almspeople were safeguarded but certain provisions were made for the admittance of future inmates. There were to be not less than twelve nor more than twenty four almspeople, to be taken as to one-half by preference, in equal numbers from Shaw-cum-Donnington and Bucklebury parishes, from persons who had resided in one of them for not less than five years, and the remainder could be from persons residing in any part of England and Wales. Those eligible for admission were poor unmarried men or women of good character of at least sixty years of age, who had not during the four years preceding their appointment received poor law relief, and who, from age, illhealth, accident or infirmity were unable to maintain themselves by their own exertions. At the same time it was stipulated that the existing hospital was to be used for male almspeople only. However, it was hoped that almshouses for twelve additional almspeople might be built when funds were available and women could then be admitted. If the patrons decided that there were no suitable persons residing in the aforesaid parishes, then, with the consent of the trustees, a person from any part of England or Wales could be appointed.

No-one was to be absent for more than twenty four hours without the written consent of the trustees or their clerk, or to part with the possession of their rooms or permit a stranger to occupy them except with special permission from the trustees. The minister had the power to make arrangements in sickness or a special emergency for the comfort of the inmates and upon the death of an existing almsman his widow had to remove from the almshouse, but the trustees were allowed to give her a pension of not more than 5s.0d. a week.

The trustees were also empowered, when income permitted, to appoint a medical officer to attend the almspeople and supply them with medicines and medical appliances at an inclusive yearly salary not exceeding £20. They could supply necessary attendance in case of illness or infirmity.

Provision was made, when funds permitted, for pensions of not less than five shillings and not more than seven shillings to be paid to poor and deserving people of not less than sixty years of age in the parishes of Shaw-cum-Donnington, Bucklebury, Iffley, Cowley, and Littlemore, providing that certain conditions were acknowledged.

Any regulations affecting the religious welfare of the recipients of the charity needed the consent of the Archbishop of Canterbury but the trustees could make other regulations consistent with the Scheme. In 1900 they drew up additional rules and provisions founded on the statutes of 1619:

1. The minister was authorised to appoint from time to time one of the almsmen to act as porter at a salary after the rate of £4 a year.
2. The almsmen were required to attend church on Sunday and festivals.
3. The almsmen were forbidden to beg.
4. The almsmen were authorised, at the discretion of the minister, to work at any manual trade within or without the hospital.
5. Provision was made for the reporting of all disputes between the almspeople to the minister, who was to decide them, or refer them to the trustees.
6. The regulation of the person appointed to attend to sick almsmen was placed in the hands of the minister.
7. No animals were to be kept.
8. The almsmen were told that it was their duty to keep their premises clean.

In 1905, upon the expiration of the term for which the representative of the minister and poor men was appointed, the trustees applied for permission to retain the services of that representative, who, being a resident of Iffley, by chance, had proved of great assistance to the trustees, and the scheme was varied accordingly.

The management of the Iffley property was placed in the hands of an estates committee of the trustees, although the minister retained the power to deal with certain small matters. The committee met monthly and were early concerned with matters relating to the drainage and water supply to the Iffley properties. The cost of repairs, improvements and rebuilding amounted to £9,300 in the eight years ending Christmas 1905, a severe drain on the income of the charity at the time, but eventually the ownership of well maintained property was to prove an asset to a charity whose income increased despite the demands of ever rising managerial expenses.

During the early years of the twentieth century the expenses of the clerk, surveyor and architect increased, also the trustees' travelling allowances, and the cost of stationery, postage and advertisements. It makes familiar reading!

In 1899 the Charity Commissioners had granted a rise in the minister's salary to £176 a year as the trustees pointed out to them that he had collected £232 more in rents during that year than in the previous one. However, when a similar plea was made in 1905 it was rejected in spite of a representation by the minister that he had visited Iffley weekly, and fortnightly collected the rents for 38 tenements, and 100 allotments. He attended the monthly meetings of the Iffley estates committee to make a return to them of the small repairs to property which he had carried out on his own responsibility, and to report to the committee the larger repairs which were necessary and needed the members' consent. Once a month he had to pay all the servants' wages as well as the allowances due to the almsmen and pensioners. He kept the accounts and rendered a monthly cash account to the trustees, and, for good measure, he held a short service in the hall of the hospital on most Sunday evenings for the almsmen, as many of them were infirm and unable to go to church.

It was agreed that the labour and time involved in these pursuits were quite considerable, but as it was deemed that both the statutes of 1393, and those of 1619, made it quite clear that the post of minister was no sinecure but one which involved unremitting labour, and that the minister did not receive less than the fee which an estate agent would expect for doing the same work, the Commissioners were not responsive and the trustees withdrew their application for a rise in the minister's salary.

A caretaker and male attendant, whose appointment was approved by the Charity Commissioners in January, 1906, occupied two rooms in the hospital, in addition to the kitchen. He received £1 weekly. This included the pay of his wife who cooked for those who were unable to carry out this task for themselves. She also acted as charwoman for the establishment but she did receive extra for this work. A housekeeper at the Iffley office received £7.16s.0d. per annum.

At that time there were twelve almsmen in residence of whom four were appointed before the 1896 scheme so that they continued to receive the stipend paid in that year, namely 25s.0d. per week for each man. The remaining eight men received 11s.6d. per week each and this included 1s.6d. for firing so that the older residents were indeed fortunate. The ages of the almsmen ranged from sixty-six to ninety-one years of age. None of them had a wife living at the hospital, but one of the pre-1896 married residents had died since that date and his widow was paid a pension of 5s.0d. a week under the terms of the scheme.

Up to 1906 it had been possible to appoint an equal number of almsmen from the parishes of Bucklebury and Shaw-cum-Donnington, but the lady of the manor of Bucklebury, Mrs Webley-Parry, and the rector of Shaw, the Rev. the Hon. John Horatio Nelson, began to experience difficulty in finding suitable applicants. This was partly due to the exclusion of married couples, and partly to the lack of poor persons in the two parishes. It is said that the two trustees had to seek out and persuade men to accept the vacancies as they occurred.

In addition to the widow already mentioned, there were sixteen out-pensioners, six in Bucklebury, two in Shaw, and eight in the Oxfordshire parishes, so that the beneficiaries became more numerous as the charity's income increased from the rise in value of its investments, and its properties in and around the expanding city of Oxford.

The Expansion of Queen Elizabeth's Hospital

Life at the hospital passed quietly during the early part of the twentieth century with some variations being made in the scheme in 1913 as experience was gained under the new administration. With the death of Mrs Webley-Parry in 1917 the hospital lost a good friend and trustee. Her Bucklebury estates passed to her younger sister, Mrs Olivia Acreman-White. In 1921 the patroness, Elizabeth Comtesse de Palatiano, died unmarried and the lordship of the manor of Donnington, and the patronage of the hospital, were inherited by her nephew, Mr Henry Hartley Aloysius Russell, the son of the late Mrs Frances Oxenham Henrietta Santa Russell, the youngest of the four heiresses.

Mr Watts continued as minister until 1932 by which time he had seen further variations made to the scheme in 1925, 1929, and April 1932. By this date the stipends of the almsmen had been raised to 15s.0d. per week, and pensions of not less than 5s.0d. and not more than £1 could be paid to other poor persons. Up to £300 a year could be given to any subsisting charities within the specified area which had for their objective the relief of the aged poor, subject to the approval of the Charity Commissioners. Also, subscriptions could be donated to any dispensary, infirmary, hospital, convalescent home, or any establishment which taught a trade to persons suffering from any bodily infirmity providing that the poor in the specified area of the charity might benefit from such instruction. Provident clubs or societies for the supply of clothing, coal, or other necessities, nursing and medical expenses, and comforts for the sick, were also entitled for consideration. Even travelling expenses for a poor patient, and the payment of contributions when a poor person could no longer continue such payments, were allowed, providing that the trustees were satisfied that the beneficiaries had shown reasonable providence. All welcome benefits before the advent of the welfare state. Mr. S. P. Inskip succeeded Mr Watts as minister and presided over the fast growing charity, under the patronage of a man who was truly concerned with the affairs of Donnington Hospital.

Mr. Henry Hartley Russell became the lord of the manor of Bucklebury in 1935 on the death of his cousin, Capt. Francis Acreman-White, and concerned himself with the welfare of the elderly residents in both his manors. In 1938 he considered the possibility of building the additional almhouses for women which had been mooted in the 1896 scheme but postponed, until the necessary funds were available. Now that the once rural area of Cowley, Iffley, and Littlemore, was becoming linked with the industrial growth of Oxford the charity could afford to build, and maintain, the additional almshouses and plans were drawn by the well known Newbury architect, Mr A. J. Campbell-Cooper, for the erection of twelve houses on a pleasant site, already owned by the Trust, in Donnington village.

The houses, which are self-contained, stand on either side of a central archway, on one side of which is the superintendent's house, and on the other a common room with a guest bedroom and bathroom overhead. The arms of Sir Richard Abberbury

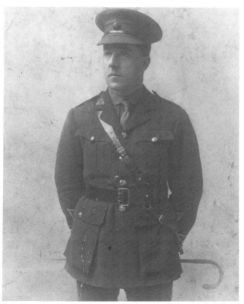

Henry Hartley Russell became Patron of the Hospital in 1921 following the death of his aunt Elizabeth, Comtesse de Palatiano

carved over the archway and the name Abberbury Close show that the fourteenth century founder was not forgotten by the twentieth century administrators of his charity when they decided to extend its services.

The builder was Mr Pembroke of Newbury, and the daughter of one of his employees used to run to watch her father at work. Today she is the wife of the present minister of the hospital.

The building cost £12,000, a sum which seems incredibly low today for the erection of such pleasant dwellings, complete with central heating and many other amenities for the comfort of the inhabitants. There was no shortage of applicants for such model almshouses. The first superintendents were Mr and Mrs H. C. Taylor.

Mr Inskip was the minister of the hospital for ten years and was succeeded by Mr Charles Bowers who held the position until 1956. Sadly his successor, Mr Cyril Bennet held office for only two years. He died in 1958 and his widow now resides in Abberbury Close. Captain Victor Byng was appointed to succeed Mr Bennet, and he was to remain as Minister for twenty five years.

The Scheme of the Charity Commissioners for the management of the hospital was revised again in 1958. The clause that 'the Owner or Owners for the time being of the Manor and Castle of Donnington shall be the Patron or Patrons of the Charity' was amended to 'the Owner or the Owners for the time being of the Manor of Donnington shall so long as the Owner is a descendant or the Owners are descendants of Frances Oxenham Henrietta Santa Russell (deceased) shall be the Patron or Patrons of the Charity'.

Another clause provided for the erection of almshouses in Iffley with the result that four very attractive flats were built in the manor which had supplied revenue for the charity over so many centuries. Hartley Russell Close stands surrounded by a lovely garden in Church Way, a reminder that near at hand is the beautiful parish church of Iffley with its wealth of Norman carving. The patron and trustees had cause to be proud of their two new additions to the charity.

A year later Donnington Hospital lost one of its most benevolent patrons. Mr Henry Hartley Russell died on Christmas Day 1959, mourned by everyone who knew him and remembered for the good work which he had done in his manors. The manors of

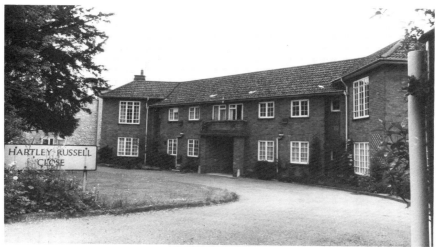

Hartley Russell Close in Church Way, Iffley. The manor of Iffley has supplied revenue for the charity over many centuries

Bucklebury and Donnington, and the patronage of the hospital, passed to his only son, Mr Derek Aylmer Hartley Russell.

The new patron sought fresh honours for the charity with a request for a grant of arms for the hospital, a request which received favourable consideration by the Earl Marshal, the Duke of Norfolk, who instructed the College of Arms to commence the necessary procedure on October 1st 1962. Mr Hartley Russell submitted his design derived from the arms of the Packers and the Hartleys: Shield – Per Fess Azure and Gules on a Fess Or between three Cross Crosslets fitchy Argent a Bar embattled Sable charged with three White Roses barbed and seeded proper.

Crest – Issuant from a Tudor Rose proper a Pelican's head and neck Or vulning herself Gules and Murally gorged Sable.

The motto was particularly appropriate – Deo et pauperibus (For God and the Poor).

The grant of arms to the Hospital of Queen Elizabeth in Donnington was signed and sealed on the twentieth day of December 1963. It was another proud day in the annals of the hospital.

However, traditional honours were not the only interest of Mr Hartley Russell. He was very much concerned with the future of the charity. The new patron foresaw that the development of

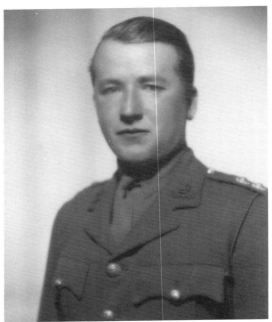

Mr Derek Hartley Russell, present Patron of the Trust

Oxford would encroach still further into the boundaries of Iffley. Already the Cowley lands of the manor had been absorbed by the expansion of the city and land at Iffley stood waiting for the next encroachment. Plans were devised whereby the land might be used for pleasing development but unfortunately the scheme ran into local opposition and was rejected by the Oxford City Council. Eventually, approximately twenty acres of land belonging to the Trust were purchased by the City Council for its own development. The patron and trustees made good use of the purchase money on behalf of the hospital.

For some years the lack of suitable dwellings for married couples had been a cause for concern. This omission was remedied in 1970 with the erection of eight modern bungalows in Bucklebury. They stand in Donnington Close at the end of a beautiful oak avenue, overlooking common land, but a village stores and post office, a butcher's shop and the Blade Bone Inn are near at hand, and buses are available to Newbury and Reading. 1983 saw four more bungalows built on an adjoining site and for these, as for all the almshouses, there is invariably a waiting list of hopeful applicants.

Other pensioners who are in need through ill-health or infirmity receive help from the charity, and societies who work for the benefit of elderly people in the appropriate manors can be sure of sympathetic consideration from the Donnington Trust which is so ably administered by the patron and trustees. Mrs Hartley Russell, the patron's wife is one of the trustees and together they take a very personal interest in the residents of the hospital.

After his long service to the charity, Captain Byng retired in 1983, and Mr R. T. Reed moved from the warden's house in Abberbury Close, together with his wife, to Bridge House, Donnington, to commence his duties as the new minister. He and the wardens of the other establishments keep a watch on the needs of the pensioners, especially if they need medical attention. Once a fortnight a minibus is available to take the residents from Donnington and Bucklebury into Newbury. This enables them to travel in comfort to make purchases which cannot be bought at the local shops. A founder's day dinner at a Newbury hotel was another thoughtful treat which was much enjoyed.

The nineteenth century report that the original almshouses in Donnington overlooked a dreary courtyard is far from the case today. All the sites have carefully tended gardens, full of colour on summer days, to add to the attractive appearance of the houses, bungalows, and flats, which make up the present day Donnington Hospital.

However, while picturesque almshouses and gardens bring admiring glances from passers-by the responsibility of the upkeep and maintenance of such properties is the continuing concern of those who administer the finances of the charity. Money must always be available for the day-to-day running expenses and for repairs and improvements, especially to the older properties. The roof of the hospital in Donnington has recently been completely overhauled, and at present plans are being prepared for a modernisation which will provide improved bathroom and toilet facilities for the twelve old almshouses.

The Trust not only invests its capital to good account, but still owns properties in the manor from which it has for so long derived its income. There are private houses in Donnington, Iffley and Cowley, a factory in Donnington, land and an hotel in Iffley, another hotel in Cowley, a cinema in Oxford, a recreation ground in Littlemore, and a farm at Sandford.

To ensure that these properties do not fall into disrepair, as has happened in the past, the Trust employs competent surveyors to supervise their repair and maintenance. The late Martin French was a most efficient surveyor. His widow still retains links with the Trust as she is now a resident of Hartley Russell Close. After Mr French's death the properties in Oxford and Iffley were placed in the care of Messrs Brooks of Oxford. It was a terrible tragedy when Robert Brooks was killed in a car accident while travelling to a meeting of the Trustees, an event which robbed them of an esteemed friend and surveyor. He was succeeded by his partner, Mr John Smith, who in turn gives valuable service by supervising the maintenance of these all-important sources of revenue. Sir Richard Abberbury, King Richard II and Queen Anne would have

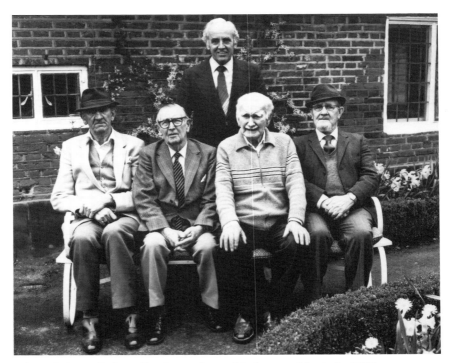

The Minister, Robert Reed together with four residents in 1985

been delighted to know that their gifts of nearly six centuries ago are still helping the poor and aged.

Since the formation of the Trust the Clerks to the Trustees have been members of the well known firm of Newbury solicitors, Messrs Pitman and Bazett. Mr Frank Bazett who served for many years is well remembered as a distinguished mayor of Newbury, and as an alderman of the Berkshire County Council. His successor, Mr Peter Faulks, held the position until his appointment as a circuit judge made it necessary for him to resign, but he was succeeded by another partner, Mr Derek Parkes, who is the present clerk and solicitor to the Trust.

The hospital has been fortunate in the choice of past and present trustees. Since the turn of the century public spirited men and women have been invited to help with the administration of the charity and they have responded by becoming involved not only in the business affairs of the hospital but also in the personal welfare of its residents.

A typical example of this type of trustee was Lt. General Callander, a distinguished soldier who lived for many years in Donnington village. He was a regular visitor to both Donnington Hospital and Abberbury Close where he enjoyed meeting the residents who regarded him as a true friend. When he left Donnington to spend his last years in Kent, he maintained his interest in the charity and regularly attended meetings of the trustees, after which he would call on his old friends before commencing his long homeward journey. No mean feat at eighty years of age.

Another faithful trustee, Mr Clifford Lovell, served for over thirty years and was elected chairman for his last year in office. He is still interested in the affairs of the hospital and its residents, many of whom he knows well, as he was a regular visitor during his many years of trusteeship.

As Mr Derek Hartley Russell looks in retrospect over the long history of his well-loved charity it is pleasing for him to think that four of the present five lay trustees are Roman Catholics as was the Founder.

In the intervening years hard times have befallen the hospital. Maladministration, and the ravages of civil war have almost destroyed it, but always a benefactor has been at hand to revive the spirit of charity and with it the life of the hospital. It stands today, extended and more prosperous than Sir Richard Abberbury could ever have envisaged. But more important than material gains, the welfare of the inhabitants is in the hands of caring trustees, minister, and wardens, while the concern of the present patron can rarely, if ever, have been surpassed in the long history of Donnington Hospital.

Lords of the Manor of Donnington

Before	1066	Toti, a Saxon.
	1066	William I.
	1086	William Lovet.
	1166	Gervasse de Salnerville.
	1229	Phillip de Salnerville.
	1231	Richard de Coupeland.
	1287	Alan de Coupeland.
	1287	Thomas de Abberbury.
	1307	Walter de Abberbury.
	1315	Richard de Abberbury.
	1333	John de Abberbury.
	1553	Sir Richard de Abberbury.
after	1397	Richard de Abberbury.
	1415	Thomas Chaucer.
	1434	William de la Pole, Earl (later Duke) of Suffolk.
	1450	John de la Pole, Duke of Suffolk.
	1491	Edmund de la Pole, Earl of Suffolk. (attainted 1503)
	1503	Henry VII. (by forfeiture)
	1509	Henry VIII.
	1514	Charles Brandon, Duke of Suffolk.
	1535	Henry VIII.
	1547	Edward VI.
	1551	The Lady Elizabeth (afterwards Queen Elizabeth I)
	1600	Charles Howard, Earl of Nottingham.
	1615	Lady Anne Howard of Effingham (later together with her son-in-law, John Mordaunt, Earl of Peterborough)
	1632	John Packer.
	1649	Robert Packer.
	1681	John Packer.
	1682	Robert Packer.
	1731	Winchcombe Howard Packer.
	1746	Henry John Packer.
	1746	Winchcombe Henry Hartley
	1794	Rev. Winchcombe Henry Howard Hartley.
	1832	Col. Winchcombe Henry Howard Hartley.
	1881	Elizabeth, Comtesse de Palatiano. (until 1906 jointly with her three sisters.)
	1921	Henry Hartley Aloysius Russell.
	1959	Derek Aylmer Frederick Henry Howard Hartley Russell.

Ministers of the Hospital from the Year 1500

1500 Robert Harre.
1509 Winston Browne.
1509 Sir John Daunce.
1513 Sir William Compton.
1514 Edward Fettiplace.
1559 Thomas Carradine.
1561 Thomas Beke.
1567 Thomas Litherland.
1597 Sir Anthony Ashley.
1599 Thomas Flory.
1601 John Duke.
1608 Richard James.
1643 Humfrey Sutton.
1644 Richard Lawrence.
1652 Walter White.
1686 Ralph Saunders.
1733 John Descrambes.
1738 William Law.
      Walter Law. (appointed some time before 1802)
1814 Joseph Edge.
1826 Thomas Nalder.
1865 Charles Graham.
1877 George Beckhuson.
1881 George Watts.
1932 S. P. Inskip.
1942 Charles Bowers.
1956 Cyril Bennet.
1958 Victor Byng.
1983 Robert Reed.

Index

ACKNOWLEDGEMENTS

An ambition was realised when Mr. Derek Hartley Russell asked me to write the history of Donnington Hospital. I had been fascinated by the charity for many years and was thrilled to have the opportunity of researching into its long history.

I would like to thank Mr. Hartley Russell for entrusting this task to me and for permission to use his family records. Also to his son, Robin Hartley Russell, for his interest and help with the research. Other information has been gathered from the Public Record Office, the Berkshire Record Office, and the Transactions of the Newbury District Field Club.

My thanks, too, to Nicholas and Suzanne Battle of Countryside Books and their staff, for assistance in the publication of the history, and the admirable photographs which illustrate the book.